DIABETIC AIR FRYER COOKBOOK #2020

Easy and Healthy Diabetic Recipes for Your Air Fryer with 30-Days Meal Plan

AMZ PUBLISHING

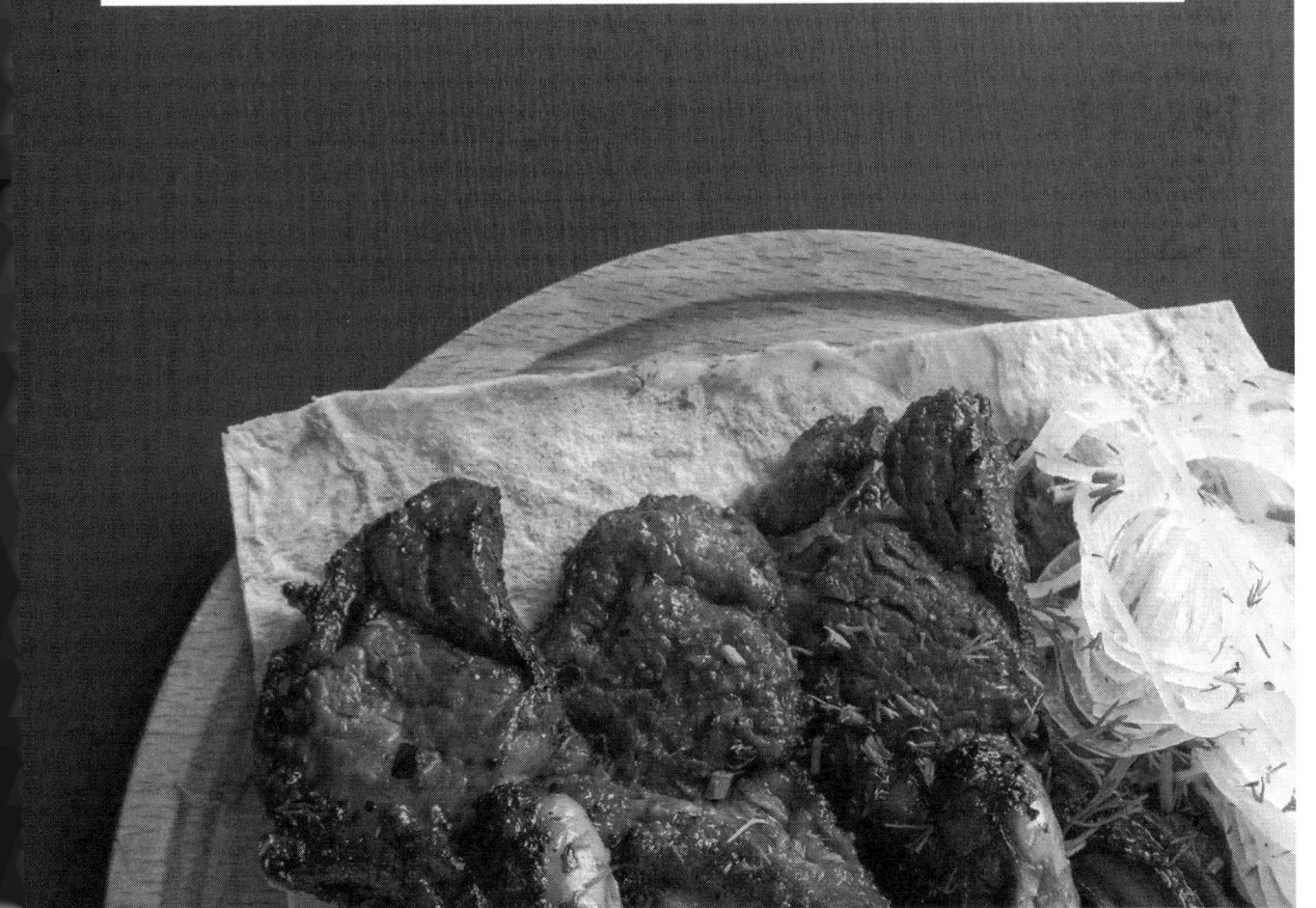

TABLE OF CONTENTS

Introduction — 4

- What is diabetes? - 5
- Types of Diabetes, Symptoms, and Treatment - 7
- Understanding the Air Fryer - 12
- How to Start Cooking in an Air Fryer - 11

30-Days Meal Plan — 14

Breakfast Recipes — 17

- Air-Fried Crispy Egg Cups - 18
- Air Fryer Scrambled Eggs - 20
- Egg Fry in an Air Fryer - 22
- Egg-Stuffed Bell Peppers - 24
- Frittata in an Air Fryer - 26
- Low-Carb Cheese, Egg, and Bacon Roll - 28
- Low-Carb Scotch Eggs in an Air Fryer - 30

Poultry Recipes — 33

- Air-Fried Buffalo Chicken Wings - 34
- Asian-Style Low-Carb Meatballs - 36
- Classic Chicken Thighs in an Air Fryer - 38
- Crispy Low-Carb Fried Chicken - 40
- Sesame Chicken Thighs - 42
- Turkey Breast in an Air Fryer - 44

TABLE OF CONTENTS

Beef, Pork, and Lamb Recipes — 47

- Air-Fried Beef Meatloaf- 48
- Air-Fried Bun Thit Nuong - 50
- Beef Satay in an Air Fryer - 52
- Cumin and Sichuan Lamb - 54
- Flank Steak Topped with Zhoug - 56
- German-Style Rouladen - 58
- Lamb Sirloin Steaks in an Air Fryer - 60
- Pork Chops in an Air Fryer - 62

Vegetarian Recipes — 65

- Air-Fried Eggplant Pizza - 66
- Chermoula Air-Fried Beets - 68
- Crispy Buffalo Cauliflower - 70
- Crisped Tofu in an Air Fryer - 72
- Easy-Peasy Ratatouille -74
- Healthy Brussels Sprouts - 76
- Low-Carb Lebanese Muhammara - 78
- Stuffed Cremini Mushrooms – 80

Seafood Recipes — 83

- Air Fryer Fish En Papillote - 84
- Air-Fried Shrimp Scampi - 86
- Cheesy Crab Dip - 88
- Healthy Niçoise Salad - 90
- Low-Carb Bok Choy Salmon - 92
- Scallops in Creamy Tomato Basil Sauce - 94

INTRODUCTION

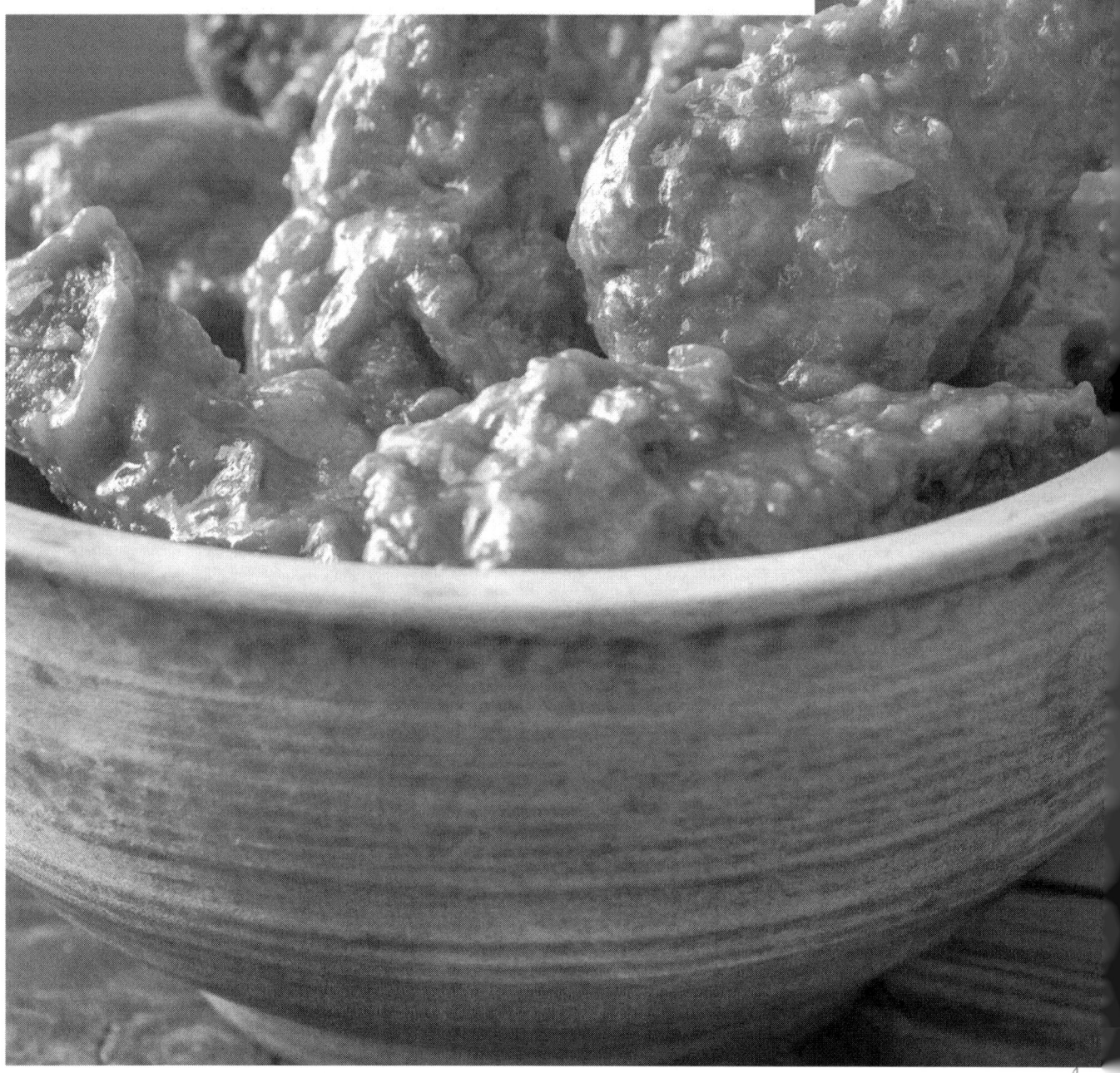

UNDERSTANDING DIABETES

Essential to the development of the human body, blood glucose acts as our main source of energy.

However, an excess of the same blood sugar levels makes the body function abnormally, resulting in diabetes.

In the case of a diabetic patient, the insulin produced by the pancreas, responsible for breaking down glucose in your body to be used for energy, is either no longer produced or is not produced in a sufficient quantity, therefore preventing glucose from reaching your cells.

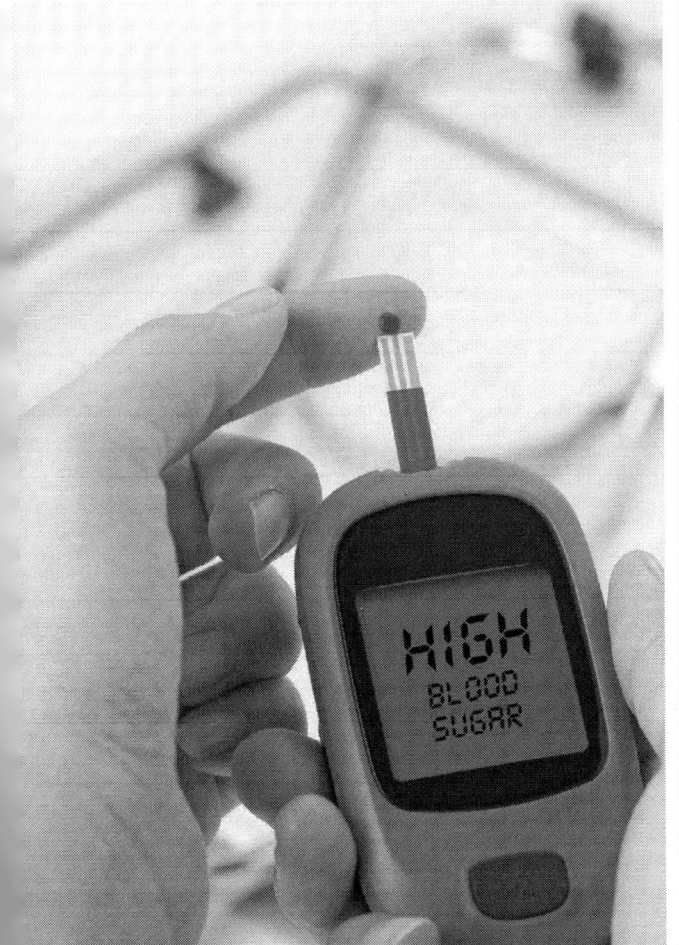

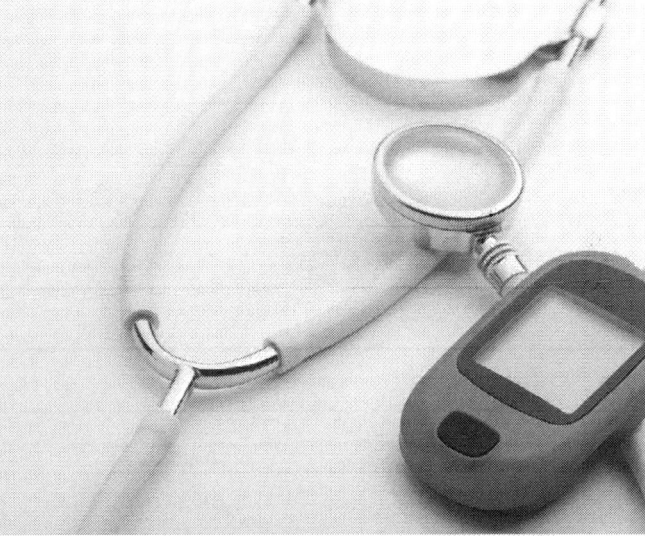

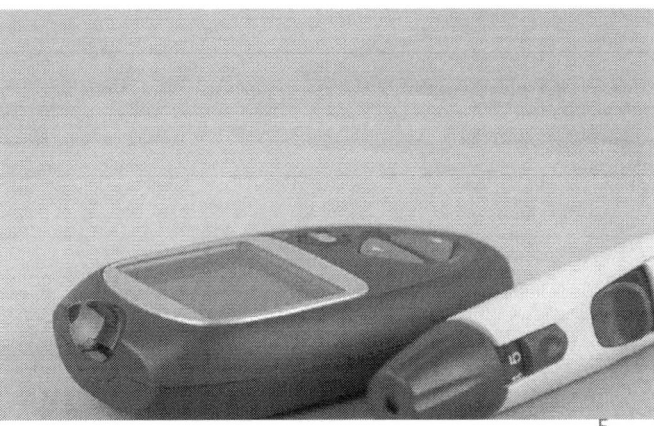

The excess of glucose thus stays in your blood and causes health problems. Though diabetes is not treatable, calculated diagnosis can help you prevent the disease, as well as keep the harm done by the disease to a minimum.

Diabetes is fast becoming one of the most common diseases today. While it used to affect primarily people over 35 years old, diabetes is now commonly seen in kids and young adults.

One of the reasons for this shift is the unhealthy lifestyle and lack of physical activity among youngsters. Our fast-paced lives have left us fixated on packaged food and engaging in minimal physical activity. Highly processed food shoots blood sugar to an abnormal level, resulting in the early onset of diabetes.

Diabetes can have an adverse effect on your body if left untreated. The disease tends to particularly attack the heart and vascular system. This may cause various heart ailments, stroke, kidney disease, or partial blindness, among other serious health hazards.

The best remedy when you are diagnosed with diabetes is to consult a doctor, seek professional help, and conduct an absolute makeover of your unhealthy lifestyle

TYPES OF DIABETES, SYMPTOMS, AND TREATMENT

Based on the condition, diabetes can be of three types:

1. Type 1 Diabetes
2. Type 2 Diabetes
3. Gestational Diabetes

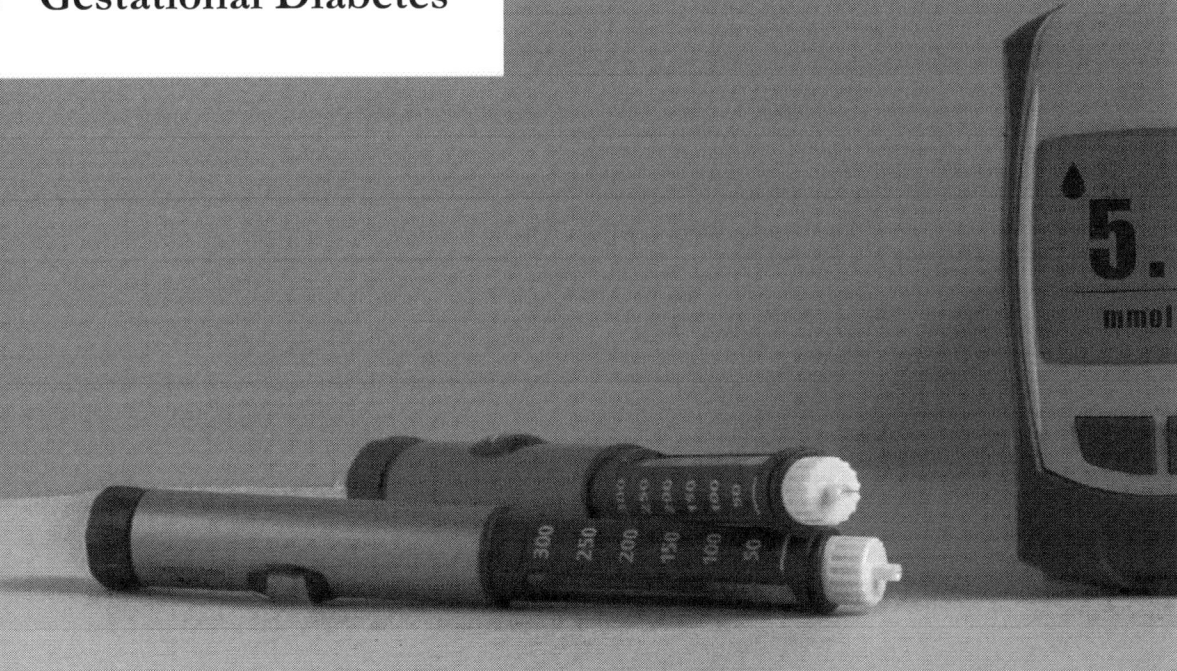

WHAT IS TYPE 1 DIABETES?

Based on the condition, diabetes can be of three types:

This is the most advanced of them all. Type 1 diabetes can be found in both children and adults. It is sometimes referred to as juvenile diabetes. This state refers to the condition in which the body of the patient stops making insulin. Without insulin, blood sugar shoots to abnormal levels and weakens the immune system.

The patient suffering from Type 1 diabetes must be administered with insulin through external sources every day of their life. The patient must also follow a controlled diet and engage in physical exercise throughout their life. Complications such as stroke, kidney failure, diabetic ketoacidosis, nonketotic hyperosmolar coma, and heart disease are common to patients suffering from Type 1 diabetes.

Symptoms include extreme thirst, more-than-usual urination, unexplained weight loss, blurring of vision, low immune system, fatigue, dry/itchy skin, and swollen or tender gums.

TREATMENT: The disease is incurable. The patient must receive insulin shots, take medication, follow a controlled diet, and engage in physical exercise.

WHAT IS TYPE 2 DIABETES?

One of the most common types of diabetes, this is a condition in which the body of the patient is producing less or not enough insulin to function normally.

The patient suffering from Type 2 diabetes has a high blood sugar level but does not need to be administered with insulin for life support. This occurs because the cells of the patient fail to respond to insulin secreted by the pancreas. The patient must consult a doctor, take medication, and change their eating and lifestyle habits.

SYMPTOMS: The symptoms of Type 2 diabetes are not as easily visible as those of Type 1 diabetes. The person can get timely checkups to determine their blood sugar level.

Treatment: The patient must begin exercising regularly and maintain a healthy diet and body mass index. If the patient is not able to suppress blood sugar levels, the doctor might prescribe medication.

WHAT IS GESTATIONAL DIABETES?

In the case of gestational diabetes, a woman, either during pregnancy or just after pregnancy, develops high blood sugar levels.

The disease may vanish after the pregnant woman delivers her child, though one must be careful to treat the patient well during the pregnancy period.

In certain cases, when a mother with gestational diabetes delivers her child, the newborn may suffer from low blood sugar or jaundice.

PRECAUTIONS: The woman must stick to a very healthy lifestyle during pregnancy.

An Appeal from the Publisher

Hello wonderful reader!

We hope you are enjoying this book.

We wanted to let you know that you have made an impact on many lives by purchasing this book.

Just to give you a brief introduction: We are a small publishing company with a team of 8 writers and 2 editors.

Most of our employees come from financially weaker section and our company is the only means they support their families. This is our way of giving back to the society.

We don't have the giant advertising budgets that many other publishers and businesses do online.

So, one way that you can really support our mission and our business is by leaving us a review on this book.

For a small company like us, getting reviews (especially on Amazon) means we can submit our books for advertising.

This means we can actually sell a few copies from time to time and make a bigger impact on the society as a whole. So, every review means a lot to us.

We can't THANK YOU enough for this!

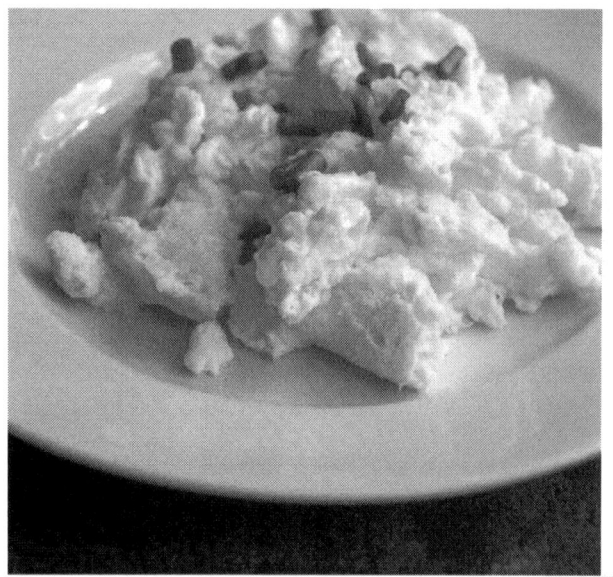

UNDERSTANDING THE AIR FRYER

A mini version of a convection oven, an air fryer is a kitchen appliance that helps you fry food without using oil. An air fryer uses the convection mechanism to fry food items by circulating hot air around the food.

It brings several benefits to the table, especially for people with specific needs, such as diabetics. The machine promotes healthy eating without compromising on taste.

Food prepared in an air fryer is not only delicious but looks just like food fried in oil, minus the harmful calories. Grill, roast, bake, fry: name it and the air fryer can handle it in a jiffy.

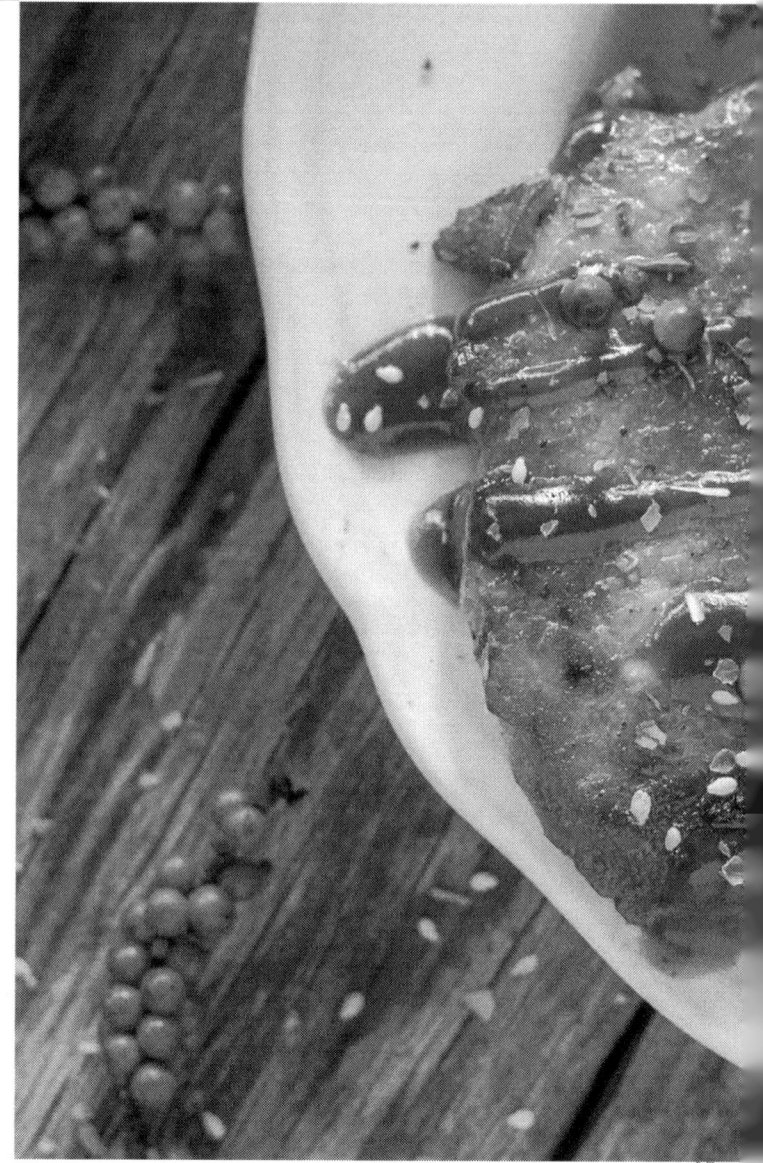

How to Start Cooking in an Air Fryer?

There is a reason why this cookbook is dedicated to recipes for people dealing with diabetes. We do not want you to have to give up on your taste buds to prevent the ailment.

Cooking in the air fryer is as easy as it gets. The revolutionary product lets you enjoy great-tasting food while keeping you on track. Just keep a few steps in mind and you are good to go.

- Always remember to place the air fryer on a heat-resistant surface, away from walls.
- Do not overload the air fryer, as it needs space to breathe.
- Depending on the workload, look for the appropriate size.
- Clean your air fryer after use.
- Do not grease the pan with cooking spray.
- Read the manual.

30-Days Meal Plan

Day	Breakfast	Lunch	Dinner
1	Frittata in an Air Fryer	Easy-Peasy Ratatouille	Classic Chicken Thighs in an Air Fryer
2	Egg-Stuffed Bell Peppers	Air-Fried Buffalo Chicken Wings	Healthy Niçoise Salad
3	Low-Carb Scotch Eggs in an Air Fryer	Air Fryer Fish En Papillote	Air-Fried Bun Thit Nuong
4	Egg Fry in an Air Fryer	Crisped Tofu in an Air Fryer	Asian-Style Low-Carb Meatballs
5	Air Fryer Scrambled Eggs	Flank Steak Topped with Zhoug	German-Style Rouladen
6	Low-Carb Cheese, Egg and Bacon Roll	Sesame Chicken Thighs	Healthy Brussels Sprouts
7	Egg-Stuffed Bell Peppers	Chermoula Air-Fried Beets	Pork Chops in an Air Fryer
8	Air Fryer Scrambled Eggs	Cheesy Crab Dip	Air-Fried Beef Meatloaf
9	Egg-Stuffed Bell Peppers	Crispy Buffalo Cauliflower	Lamb Sirloin Steaks in an Air Fryer
10	Low-Carb Scotch Eggs in an Air Fryer	Pork Chops in an Air Fryer	Beef Satay in an Air Fryer
11	Low-Carb Cheese, Egg and Bacon Roll	Air-Fried Shrimp Scampi	Stuffed Cremini Mushrooms
12	Air-Fried Crispy Egg Cups	Crispy Low-Carb Fried Chicken	Scallops in Creamy Tomato Basil Sauce
13	Frittata in an Air Fryer	Air-Fried Eggplant Pizza	Cumin and Sichuan Lamb
14	Egg-Stuffed Bell Peppers	Turkey Breast in an Air Fryer	Low-Carb Lebanese Muhammara
15	Low-Carb Scotch Eggs in an Air Fryer	Flank Steak Topped with Zhoug	Low-Carb Bok Choy Salmon

Day	Breakfast	Lunch	Dinner
16	Egg Fry in an Air Fryer	Crispy Buffalo Cauliflower	Classic Chicken Thighs in an Air Fryer
17	Air Fryer Scrambled Eggs	Easy-Peasy Ratatouille	Healthy Niçoise Salad
18	Low-Carb Cheese, Egg and Bacon Roll	Air-Fried Buffalo Chicken Wings	Air-Fried Bun Thit Nuong
19	Air-Fried Crispy Egg Cups	Air Fryer Fish En Papillote	Asian-Style Low-Carb Meatballs
20	Low-Carb Scotch Eggs in an Air Fryer	Crisped Tofu in an Air Fryer	German-Style Rouladen
21	Low-Carb Cheese, Egg and Bacon Roll	Flank Steak Topped with Zhoug	Healthy Brussels Sprouts
22	Air Fryer Scrambled Eggs	Sesame Chicken Thighs	Pork Chops in an Air Fryer
23	Egg-Stuffed Bell Peppers	Chermoula Air-Fried Beets	Air-Fried Beef Meatloaf
24	Frittata in an Air Fryer	Cheesy Crab Dip	Lamb Sirloin Steaks in an Air Fryer
25	Egg-Stuffed Bell Peppers	Crispy Buffalo Cauliflower	Beef Satay in an Air Fryer
26	Low-Carb Scotch Eggs in an Air Fryer	Pork Chops in an Air Fryer	Stuffed Cremini Mushrooms
27	Egg Fry in an Air Fryer	Air-Fried Shrimp Scampi	Scallops in Creamy Tomato Basil Sauce
28	Air Fryer Scrambled Eggs	Crispy Low-Carb Fried Chicken	Cumin and Sichuan Lamb
29	Low-Carb Cheese, Egg and Bacon Roll	Air-Fried Eggplant Pizza	Low-Carb Lebanese Muhammara
30	Air-Fried Crispy Egg Cups	Turkey Breast in an Air Fryer	Low-Carb Bok Choy Salmon

breakfast

RECIPES

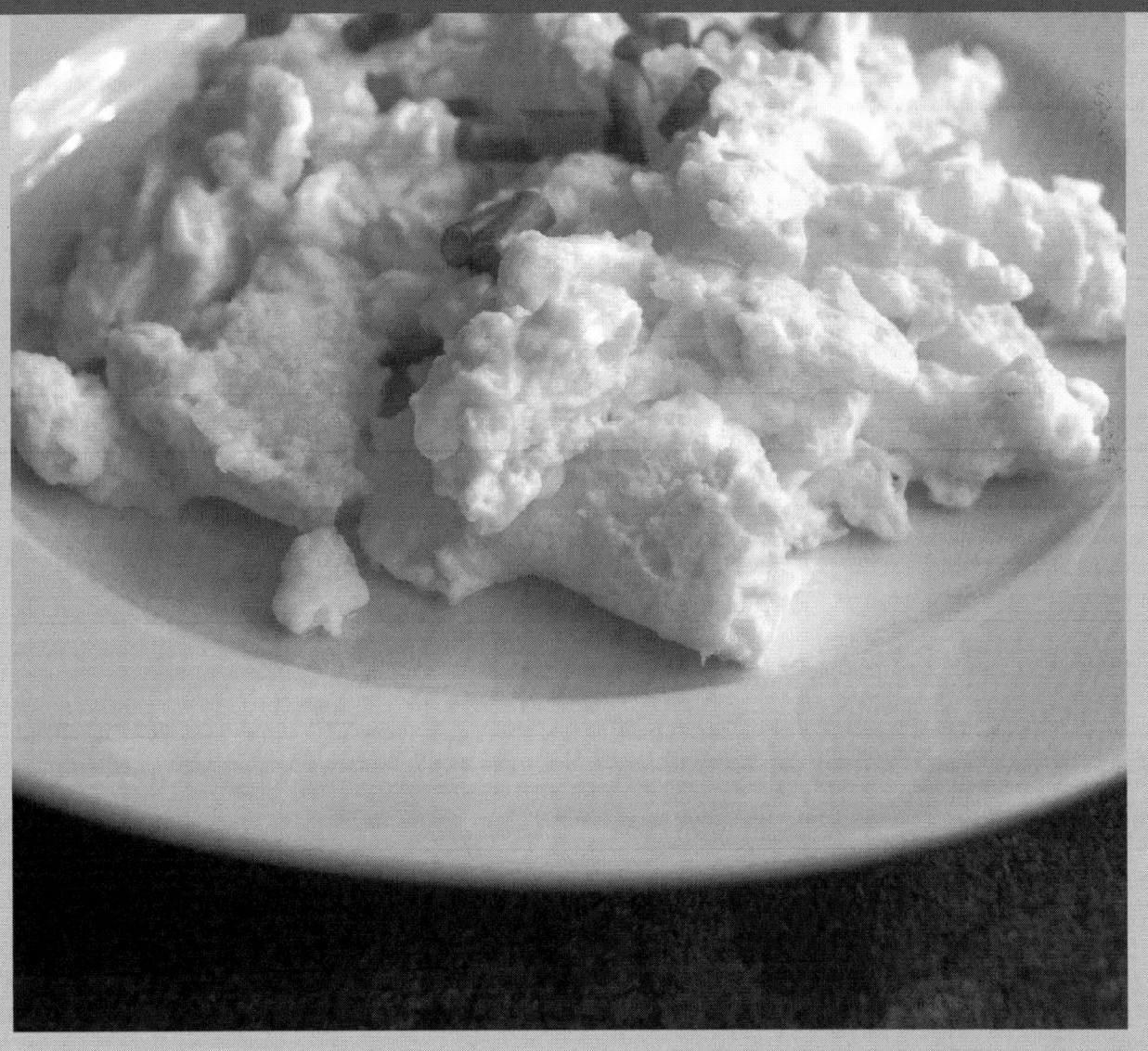

Air-Fried Crispy Egg Cups

GENERAL INFO

Serving Size: 1
Servings per Recipe: 4
Calories: 150 calories per serving
Total Time: 18 minutes

INGREDIENTS

Olive oil cooking spray
Whole wheat bread – 4 slices
Tub margarine (trans-fat-free) – 1 ½ tablespoons
Ham (deli-style) – 1 slice
Eggs – 4 large
Salt – ⅛ teaspoon
Black pepper – ⅛ teaspoon
Fresh chives (chopped) – for garnishing

NUTRITION INFO

Fat – 8 g
Protein – 12 g
Carbohydrates – 6 g

Air-Fried Crispy Egg Cups

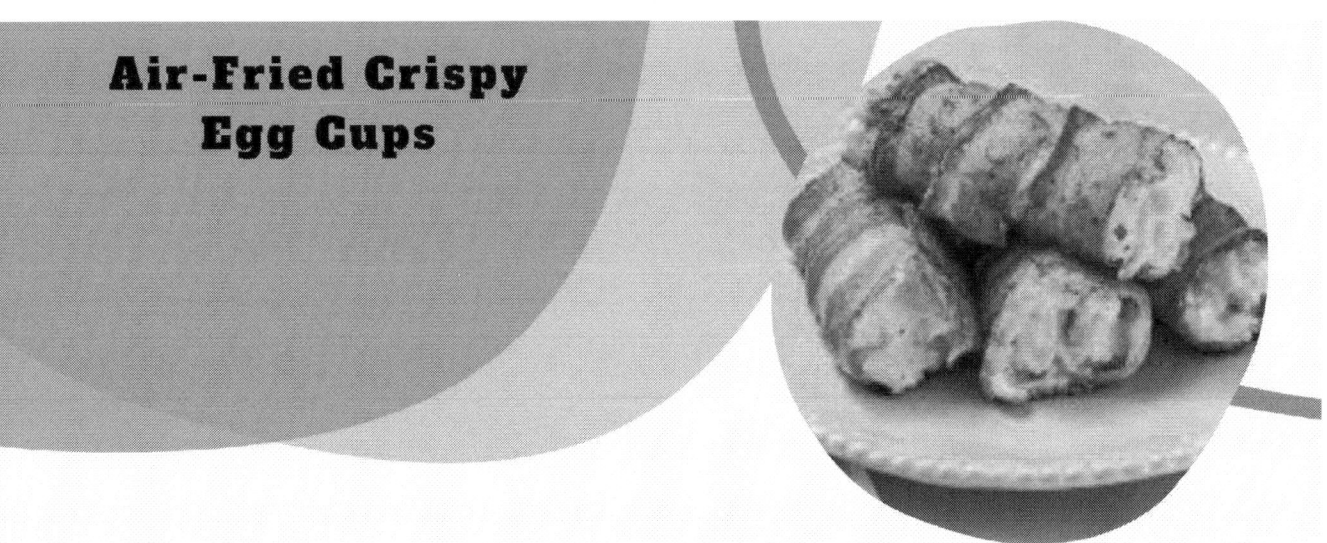

DIRECTIONS

1. Start by preheating the air fryer by setting the temperature to 375°F.
2. Slice the ham into ½-inch-thick strips.
3. Take 4 oven-safe ramekins and spray them with olive oil cooking spray.
4. Take the bread slices and lightly toast them evenly until golden brown. Cut the crust sides from the bread slices and discard.
5. Take 1 bread slice and use a butter knife to spread the margarine evenly. Place the slice into the ramekin. Make sure that the side with margarine is facing down.
6. Press the slice down to form a cup and cover evenly with ham strips.
7. Now crack an egg on top of the ham strips. Repeat the entire process with the remaining cups.
8. Finish by sprinkling the 4 slices, ham, and eggs with pepper and salt.
9. Take the basket out of the air fryer and place the prepared ramekins in the basket.
10. Let the eggs cook for about 13 minutes. The eggs should be set by now.
11. Remove the ramekins from the basket and use a knife to loosen the edges.
12. Hold the edges of the bread cups and carefully take them out of the ramekins. Place them on a serving platter.
13. Finish by garnishing with freshly chopped chives.

Air Fryer Scrambled Eggs

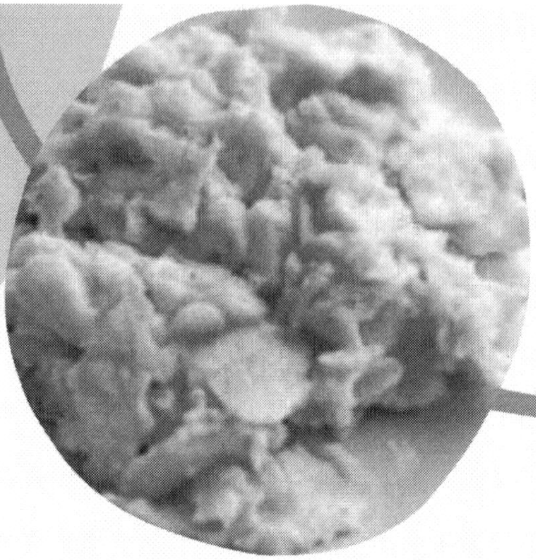

GENERAL INFO

Serving Size: 1
Servings per Recipe: 2
Calories: 188 calories per serving
Total Time: 11 minutes

INGREDIENTS

Feta cheese – 40 grams
Cayenne pepper – 1 pinch
Fresh tarragon – 5 grams
Eggs – 3 large

NUTRITION INFO

Fat – 13.7 g
Protein – 14.4 g
Carbohydrates – 1.8 g

Air Fryer Scrambled Eggs

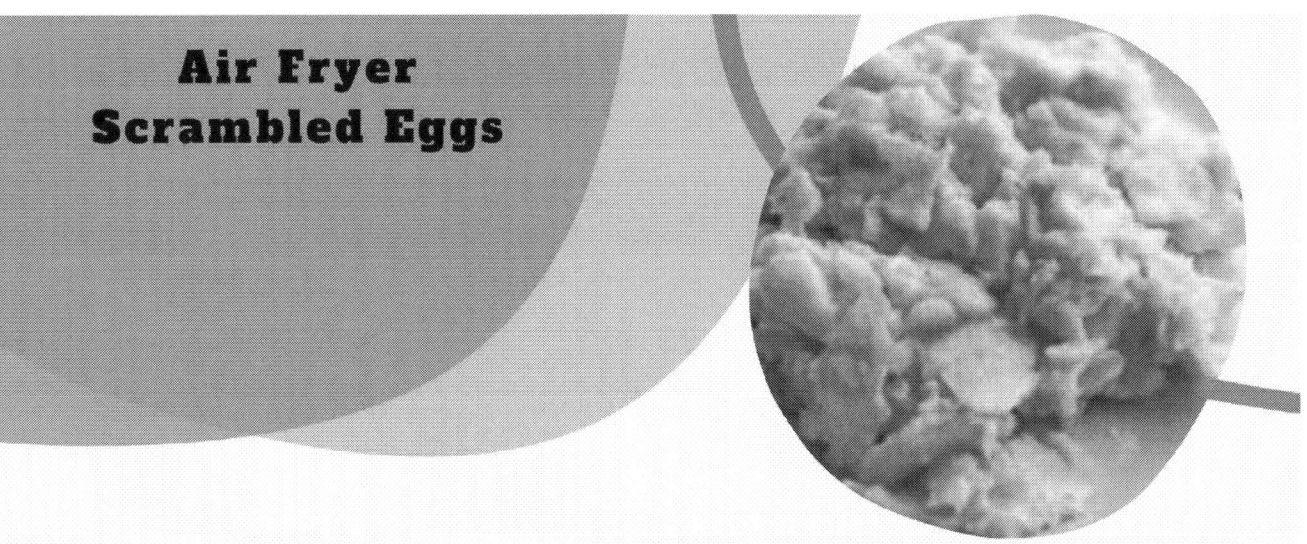

DIRECTIONS

1. Start by cutting feta cheese into bite-size cubes and finely chopping the tarragon leaves.
2. Take a bowl and crack in all the eggs. Whisk well. Transfer the whisked eggs into an aluminum tin.
3. Take the basket out of the air fryer and place the aluminum tin inside the same.
4. Start the air fryer and set the temperature to 325°F. Cook the eggs for about 3 minutes
5. Take out the basket and stir in the tarragon and feta cubes. Cook for another 3 minutes.
6. Take the basket out again and give the cheese and eggs a good stir using a spatula.
7. Return the eggs to the air fryer and cook for about 5 minutes.
8. Once done, transfer onto a serving platter and season with a pinch of cayenne pepper. Serve with a toasted bread slice.

Egg Fry

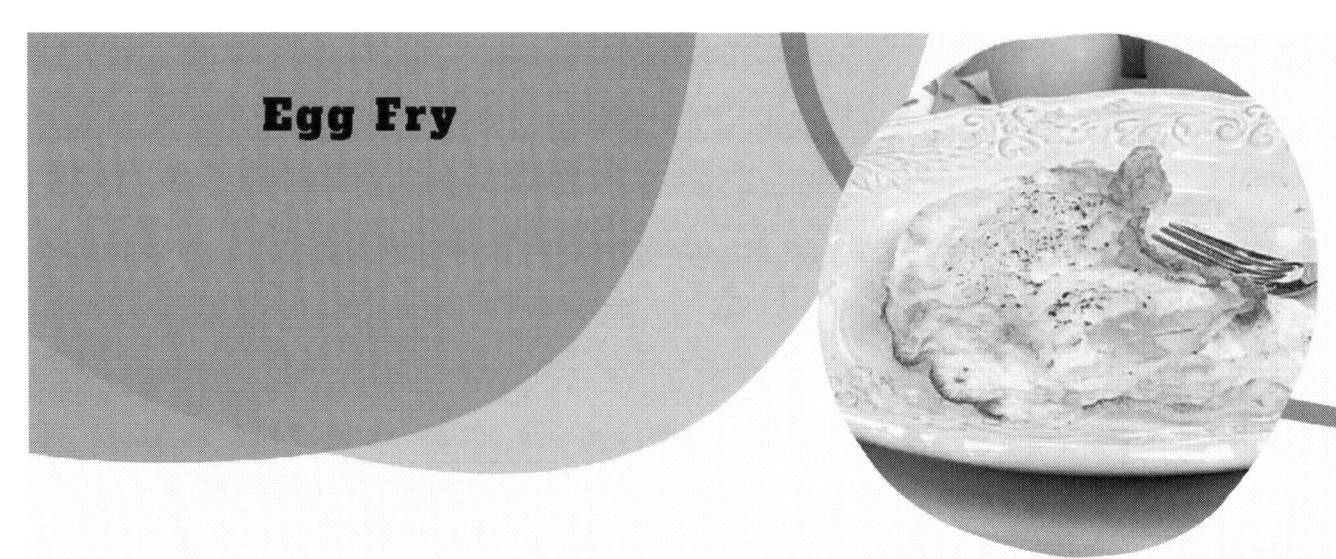

GENERAL INFO

Serving Size: 1
Servings per Recipe: 1
Calories: 363 calories per serving
Total Time: 9 minutes

INGREDIENTS

Eggs – 2 large
Butter – 2 tablespoons
Salt – as per taste
Pepper – as per taste

NUTRITION INFO

Fat – 33 g
Protein – 14 g
Carbohydrates – 1 g

Egg Fry

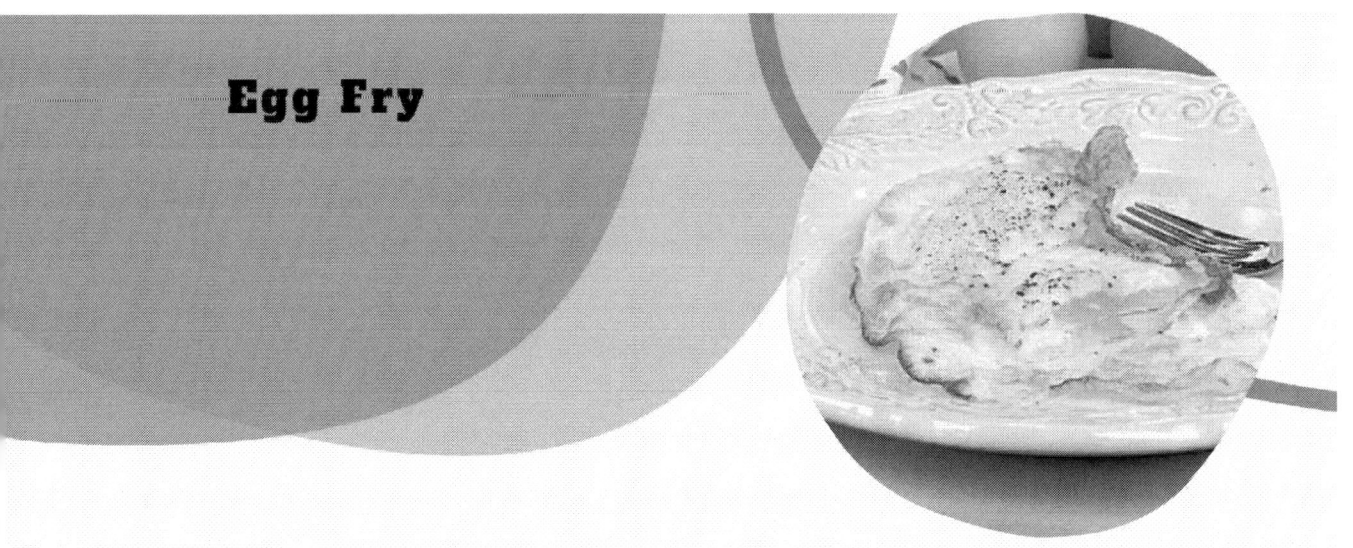

DIRECTIONS

1. Start by placing an aluminum pan into the air fryer basket.
2. Add the butter and place the basket in the air fryer. Heat the butter at 350°F until it melts completely. This should take about 1 minute.
3. Take out the basket and crack the eggs into the pan.
4. Place the basket back into the air fryer and cook for about 8 minutes at 325°F.
5. Serve hot!

Egg-Stuffed Bell Peppers

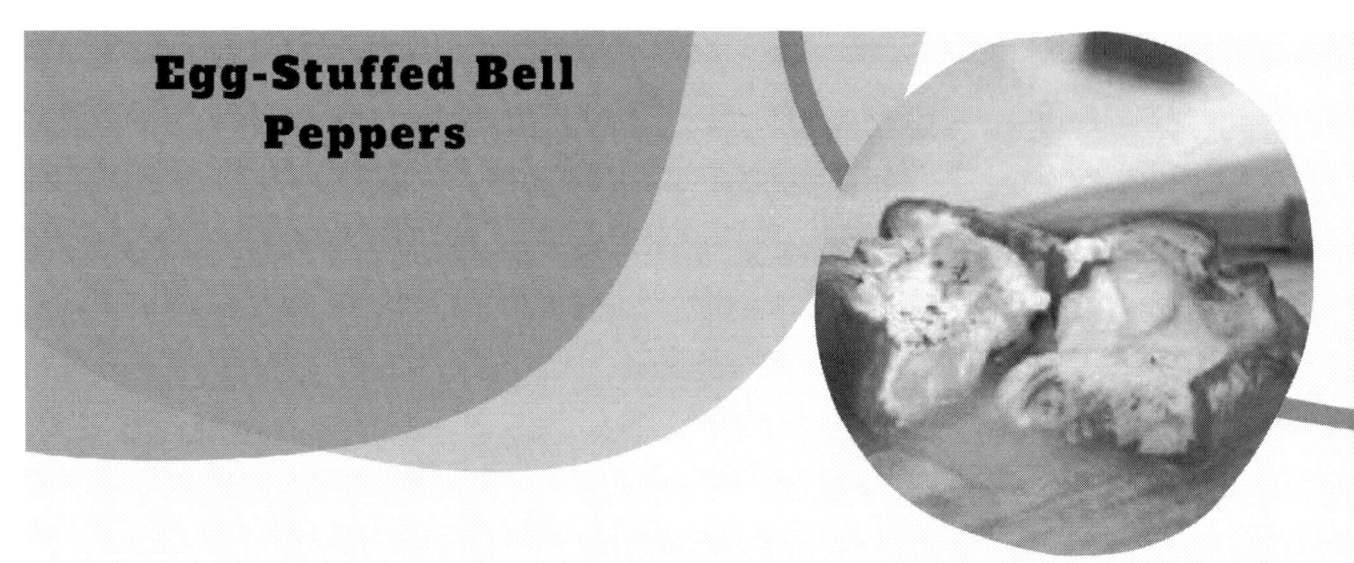

GENERAL INFO

Serving Size: 1
Servings per Recipe: 2
Calories: 164 calories per serving
Total Time: 18 minutes

INGREDIENTS

Bell pepper (deseeded and halved) – 1
Eggs – 4
Olive oil – 1 teaspoon
Salt – 1 pinch
Pepper – 1 pinch
Sriracha flakes – 1 pinch

NUTRITION INFO

Fat – 10 g
Protein – 11 g
Carbohydrates – 4 g

Egg-Stuffed Bell Peppers

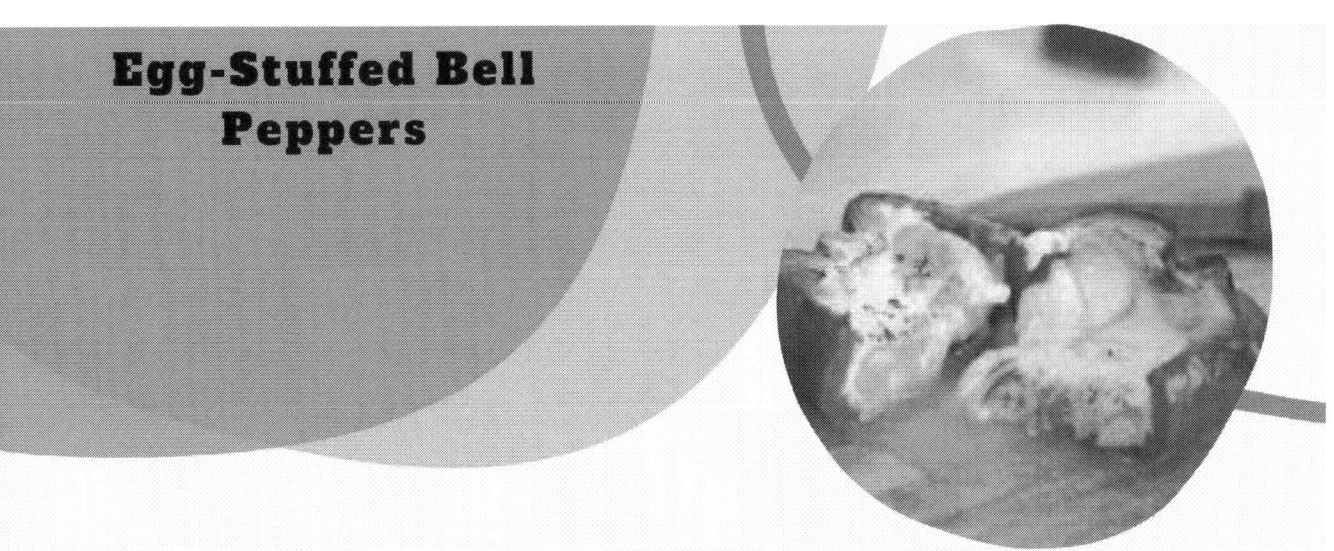

DIRECTIONS

1. Start by cutting the bell pepper through the center. Scoop out the seeds.
2. Rub the cut edges with olive oil using your finger.
3. Place the pepper halves onto a flat surface and crack 2 eggs each into both halves.
4. Generously sprinkle each of the pepper halves with salt, pepper, and sriracha flakes.
5. Take the basket out of the air fryer and place the pepper halves into the same.
6. Return the basket to the air fryer and set the timer for about 13 minutes at 390°F.
7. Take the bell peppers out of the basket and serve hot!

Frittata in an Air Fryer

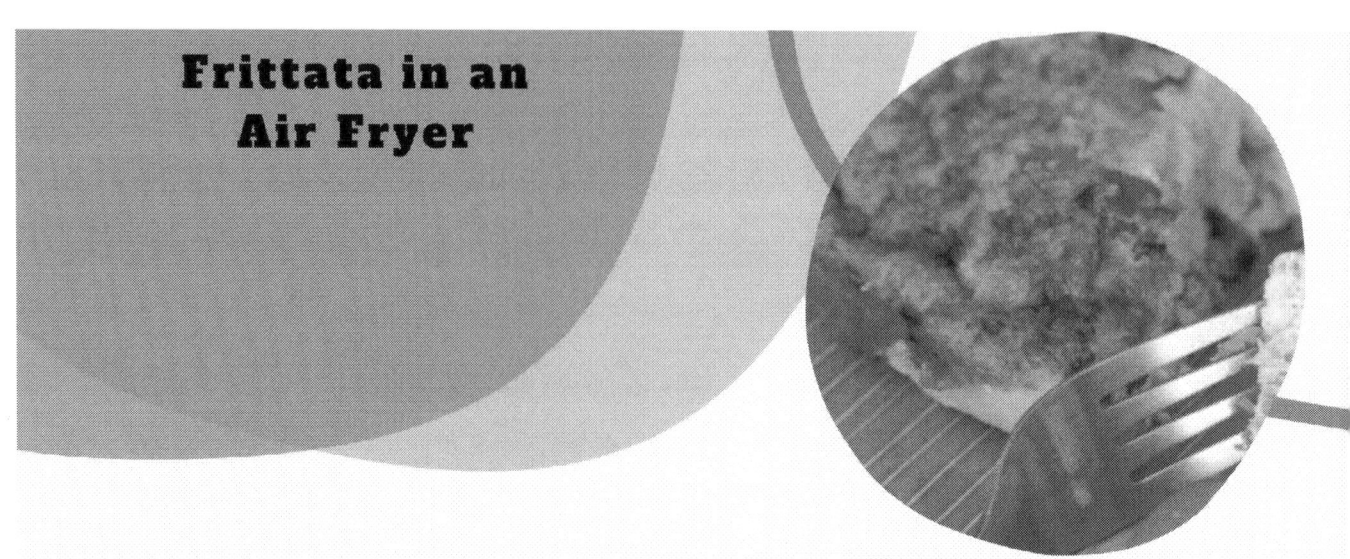

GENERAL INFO

Serving Size: 1
Servings per Recipe: 4
Calories: 190 calories per serving
Total Time: 20 minutes

INGREDIENTS

Olive oil (extra virgin) – 2 tablespoons
Sausage (chicken and sun-dried tomato sausage) – 8 ounces
Egg substitute – 1 ½ cups
Shredded mozzarella cheese (part-skim) – 1 ounce
Green onion (chopped finely) – ½ cup
Tomatoes (diced) – 1 cup
Fresh basil (chopped) – for garnish

NUTRITION INFO

Fat – 8 g
Protein – 21 g
Carbohydrates – 6 g

Frittata in an Air Fryer

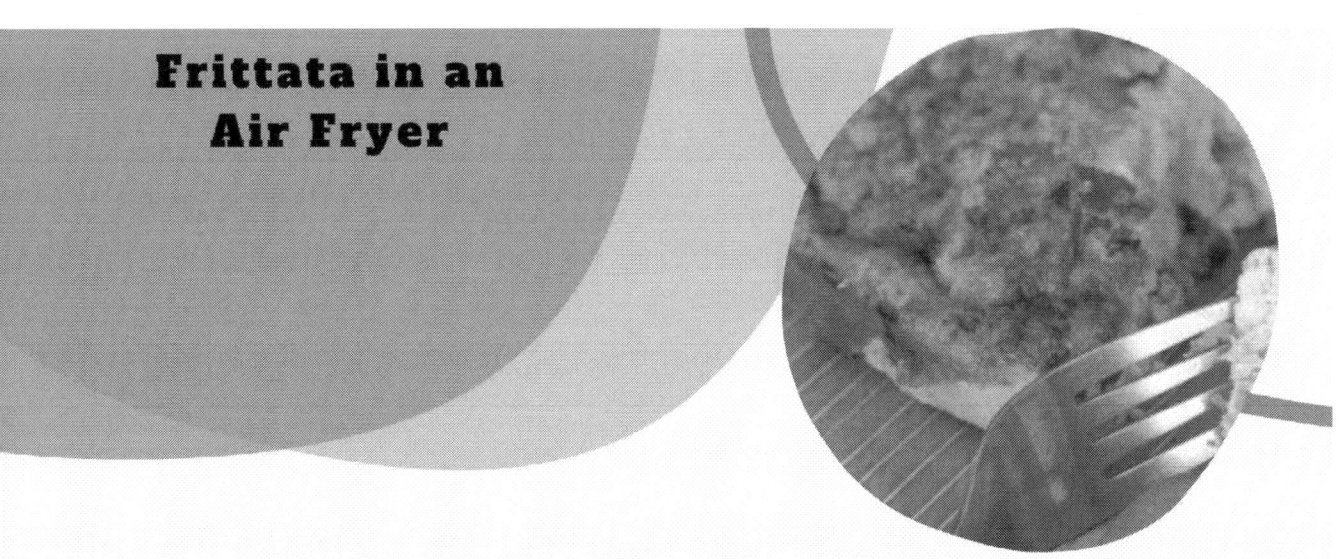

DIRECTIONS

1. Start by preheating the air fryer by setting the temperature to 320°F.
2. Dice the sausages into small pieces.
3. Take a pan and grease it using cooking spray. Place the diced sausages into the pan.
4. Remove the basket from the air fryer and place the greased pan with sausages into the same. Let them cook for about 5 minutes.
5. While the sausages are cooking, take a mixing bowl and add the egg substitute, half of the shredded mozzarella, tomatoes, and green onion. Mix well.
6. Take the pan out of the air fryer and pour in the egg substitute mixture. Cook for 10 minutes.
7. Take out the pan and spread the remaining cheese on the frittata evenly. Top with basil leaves.
8. Return the pan into the air fryer and cook for another 5 minutes.
9. Once done, cut into 4 equal-sized wedges. Serve hot!

Low-Carb Cheese, Egg, and Bacon Roll

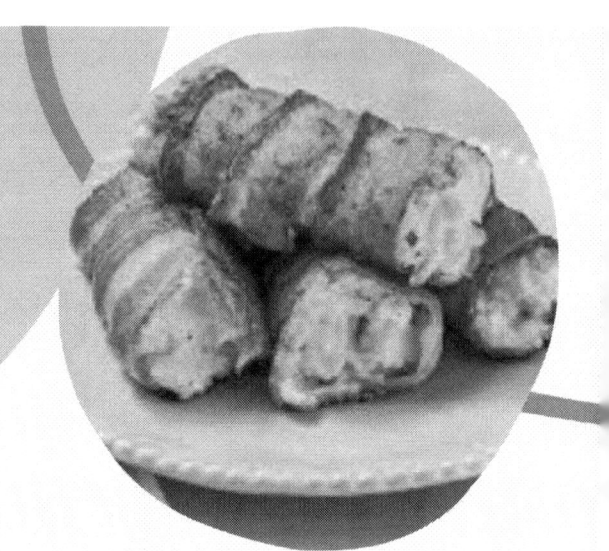

GENERAL INFO

Serving Size: 1
Servings per Recipe: 2
Calories: 680 calories per serving
Total Time: 30 minute

INGREDIENTS

Butter – 2 tablespoons
Onion (chopped) – ½ cup
Green bell pepper (chopped) – ½ cup
Eggs – 4 large
Salt – as per taste
Pepper – as per taste
Bacon (sugar-free) – 6 slices
Cheddar cheese (shredded) – ⅔ cup
Hot salsa – 1/3 cup

NUTRITION INFO

Fat – 61 g
Protein – 33 g
Carbohydrates – 9.1 g

Low-Carb Cheese, Egg, and Bacon Roll

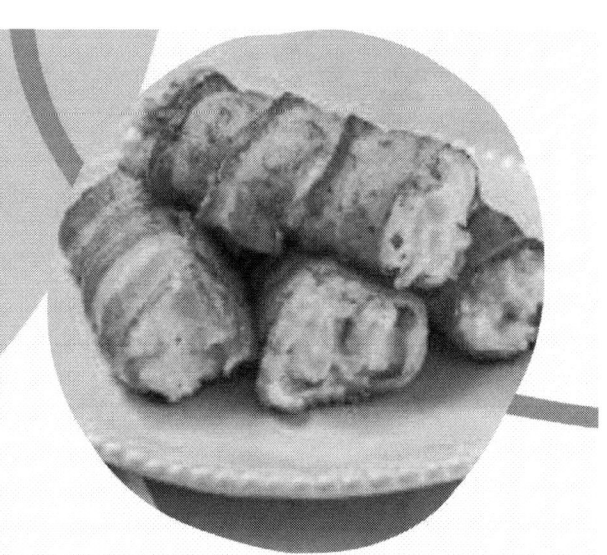

DIRECTIONS

1. Start by taking a nonstick pan and placing it over a medium flame. Add the butter and let it melt.
2. Toss the chopped onion and bell peppers into the pan. Let it cook for about 3 minutes.
3. While the veggies are cooking, take a bowl and break the eggs into the same. Whisk well and sprinkle with pepper and salt.
4. Pour the whisked eggs into the pan and let them cook for about a minute. Take off the flame and let the eggs cool down a bit. (The eggs should be set but slightly undercooked.)
5. Place the bacon slices side by side on a flat surface. Transfer half of the eggs onto the bacon slices.
6. Spread half of the shredded cheese on top of the eggs.
7. Use your hands to roll the bacon and eggs into a cylindrical shape. Secure the ends with toothpicks. Repeat the process with the remaining bacon, eggs, and cheese.
8. Place the prepared bacon rolls into the air fryer basket and cook for about 8 minutes at 350°F. Flip over and cook for another 7 minutes.
9. Once done, transfer onto a serving platter. Serve with hot salsa.

Low-Carb Scotch Eggs

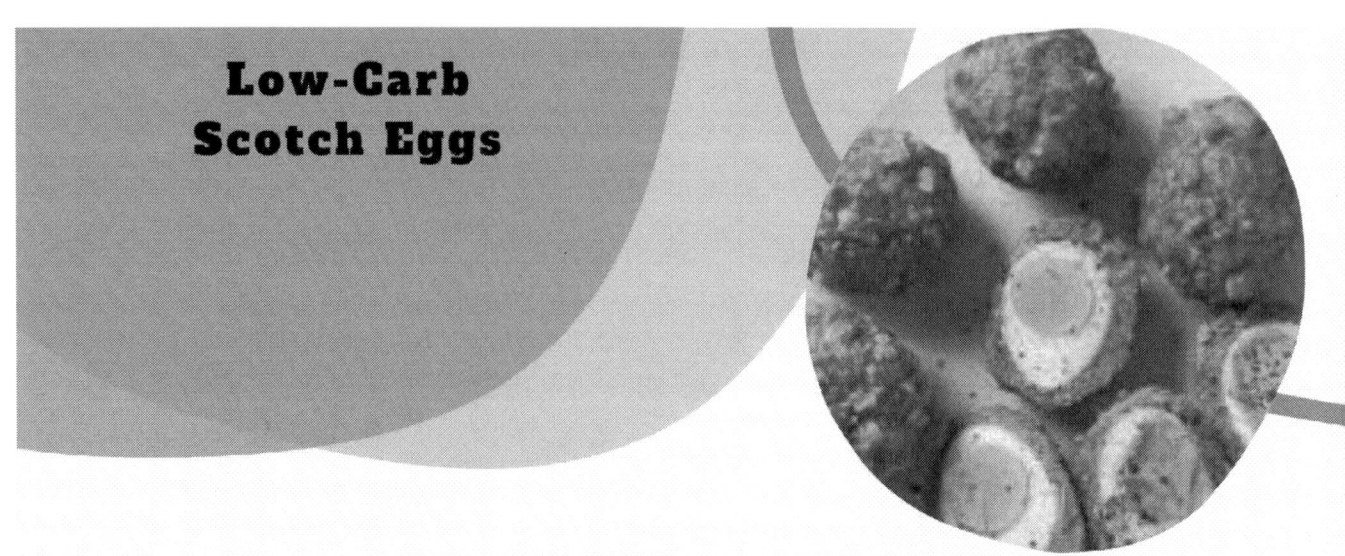

GENERAL INFO

Serving Size: 1
Servings per Recipe: 4
Calories: 506 calories per serving
Total Time: 13 minutes

INGREDIENTS

Ground breakfast sausage – 1 pound
Soft-boiled eggs – 4
Grated parmesan cheese – 1 cup
Fresh parsley (finely chopped) – 2 tablespoons

NUTRITION INFO

Fat – 40.7 g
Protein – 31.6 g
Carbohydrates – 1.25 g

Low-Carb Scotch Eggs

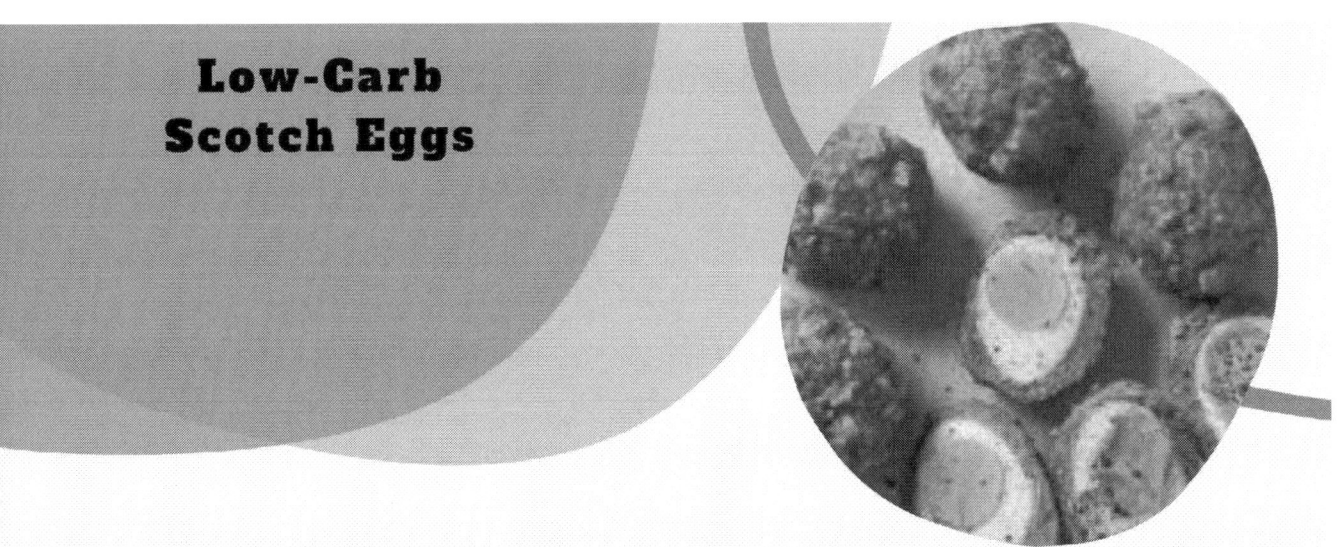

DIRECTIONS

1. Start by preheating the air fryer.
2. Take a large mixing bowl and add the ground sausage and finely chopped parsley. Use your hands to knead until well-combined.
3. Divide the pork mixture into 4 equal parts and use your hands to form a patty with each part.
4. Take 1 patty and place a soft-boiled egg in the center. Cover the egg completely with the pork patty. Repeat the process with all the remaining eggs. Make sure the eggs are perfectly coated and there are no gaps.
5. Place the grated parmesan in a shallow dish and dredge the coated eggs into the same. Make sure the eggs are evenly coated.
6. Place the prepared eggs into the air fryer basket and spray them lightly with avocado oil.
7. Let the eggs cook for about 7 minutes. Flip over and spray the other side with avocado oil. Air-fry for another 7 minutes.
8. Once done, take out of the air fryer and serve hot with Dijon mustard.

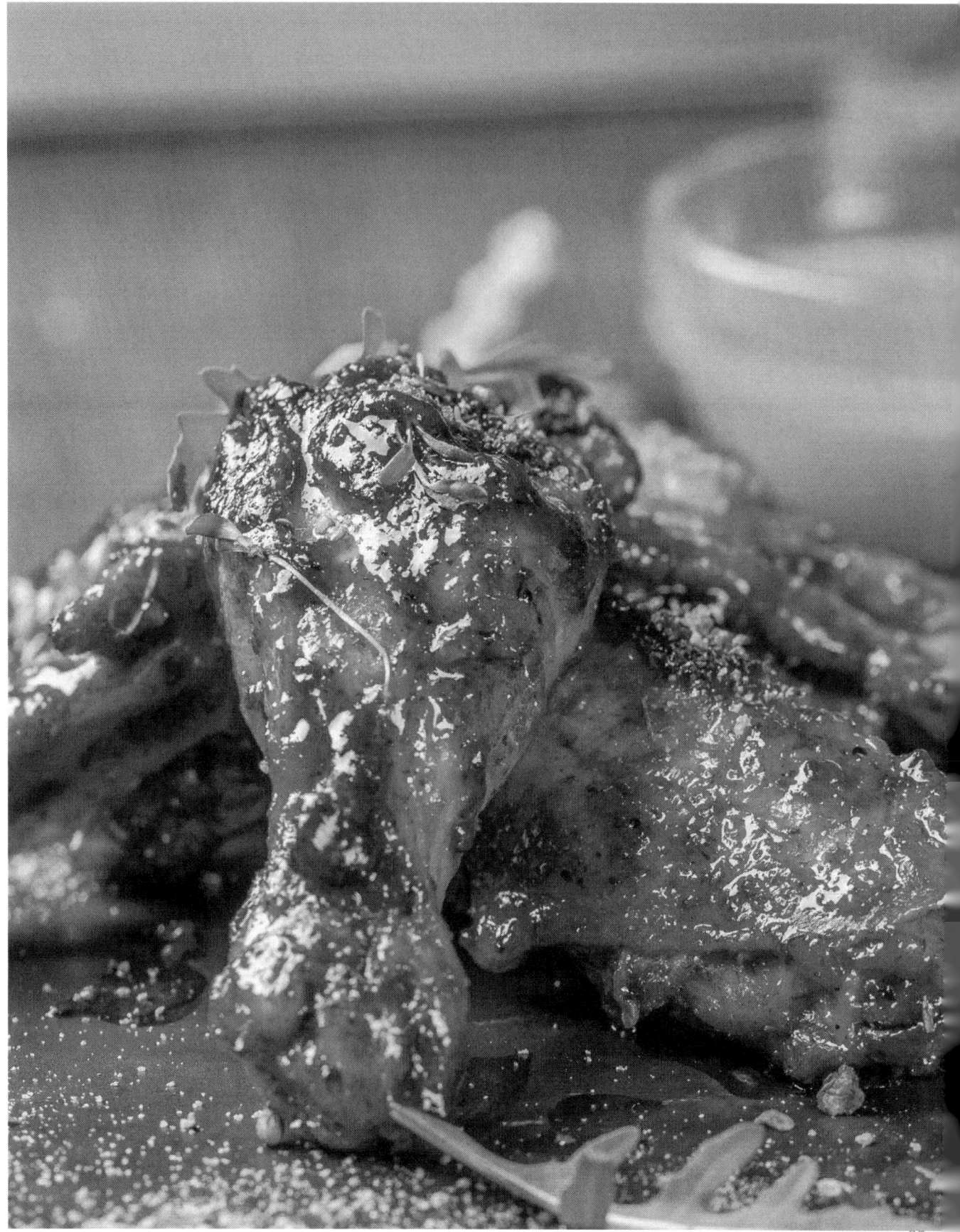

poultry
RECIPES

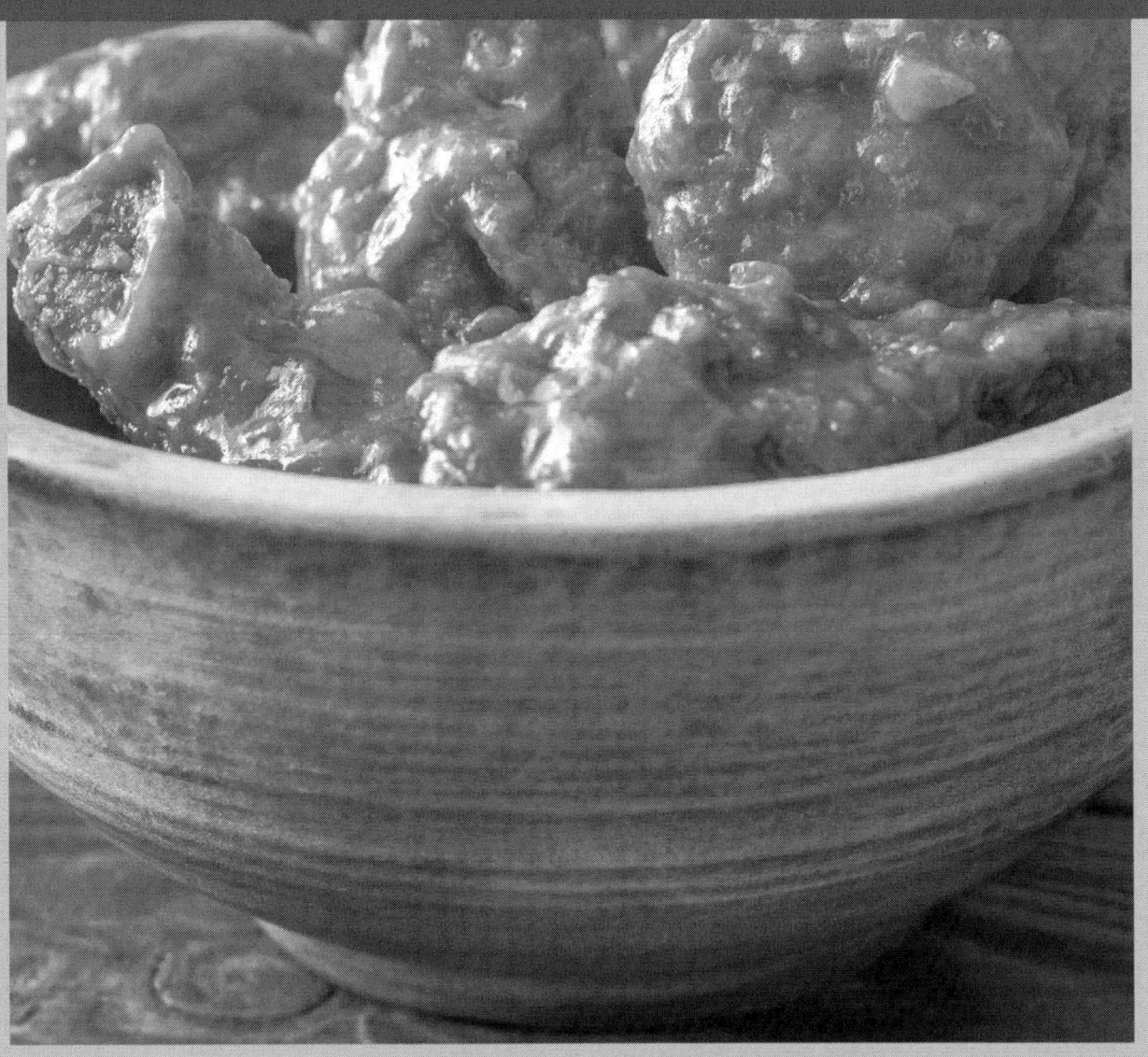

Air-Fried Buffalo Chicken Wings

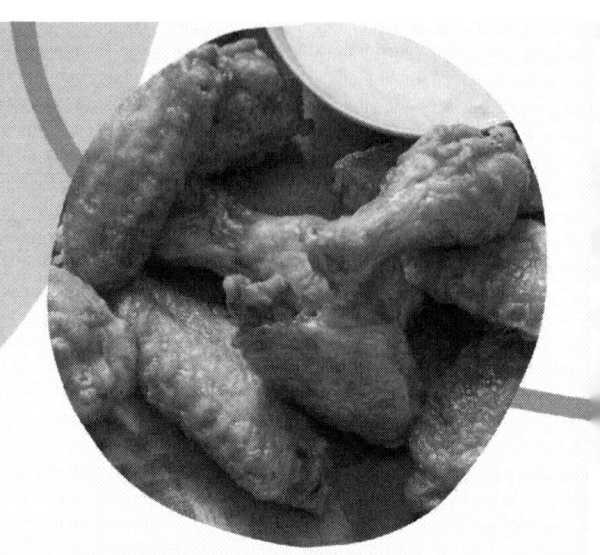

GENERAL INFO

Serving Size: 1
Servings per Recipe: 4
Calories: 481 calories per serving
Total Time: 1 hour and 5 minutes

INGREDIENTS

Chicken wings – 2 ½ pounds
Olive oil – 1 tablespoon
Cayenne pepper sauce – ⅔ cup
Butter – ½ cup
Vinegar – 2 tablespoons
Garlic powder – 1 teaspoon
Cayenne pepper – ¼ teaspoon

NUTRITION INFO

Fat – 41.5 g
Protein – 20.7 g
Carbohydrates – 7.3 g

Air-Fried Buffalo Chicken Wings

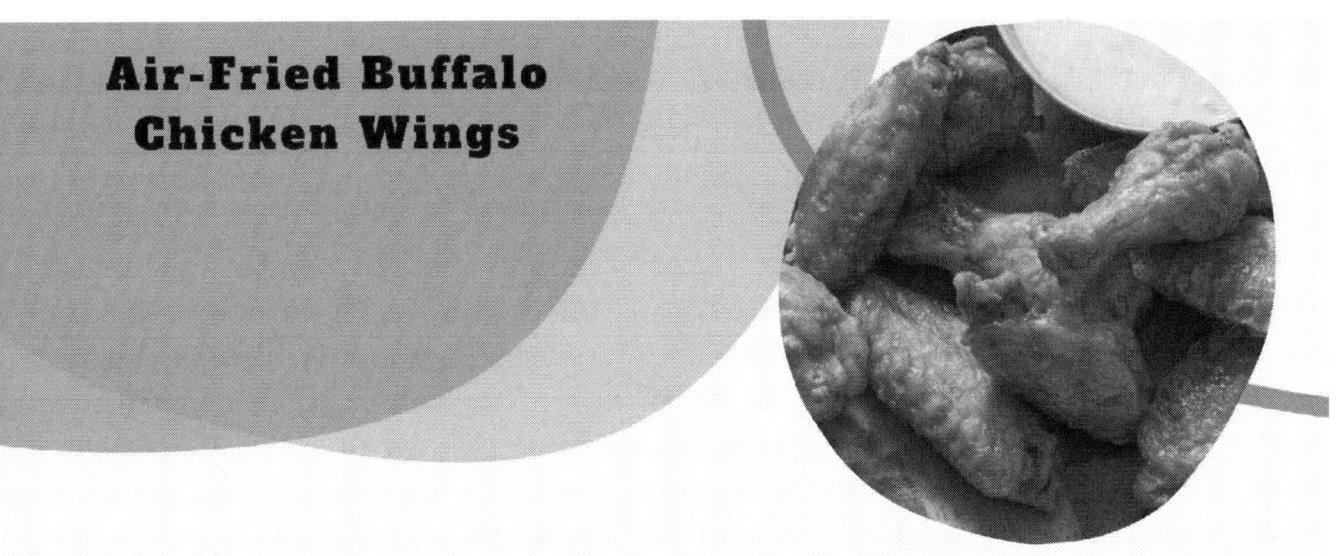

DIRECTIONS

1. Start by preheating the oven by setting the temperature to 360°F.
2. Take a large mixing bowl and add the wings. Pour in the olive oil and gently massage the chicken breasts. Make sure all the wings are evenly coated.
3. Take out the air fryer basket and place half of the chicken wings into the same. Make sure there is a little space between each of the wings.
4. Transfer the basket back into the air fryer and cook for about 25 minutes.
5. Open the basket, flip the wings, and let them cook for another 5 minutes.
6. Transfer the air-fried wings to a large glass bowl. Repeat the process with the rest of the wings.
7. While the second batch of wings is cooking, in a medium-sized mixing bowl, add the butter, cayenne pepper sauce, garlic powder, cayenne pepper, and vinegar. Mix until well-combined.
8. Once air-fried, transfer the second batch of wings into the bowl with the previously fried chicken wings.
9. Pour the prepared hot sauce over the air-fried chicken wings and mix until all the wings are evenly coated.

Asian-Style Low-Carb Meatballs

GENERAL INFO

Serving Size: 1
Servings per Recipe: 4
Calories: 223 calories per serving
Total Time: 25 minutes

INGREDIENTS

Ground chicken – 1 pound
Green onions (chopped) – 2
Cilantro (chopped) – ½ cup
Hoisin sauce – 1 tablespoon
Soy sauce – 1 tablespoon
Sriracha sauce – 1 teaspoon
Sesame oil – 1 teaspoon
Unsweetened coconut (shredded) – ¼ cup
Salt – as per taste
Black pepper (ground) – as per taste

NUTRITION INFO

Fat – 14 g
Protein – 20 g
Carbohydrates – 3 g

Asian-Style Low-Carb Meatballs

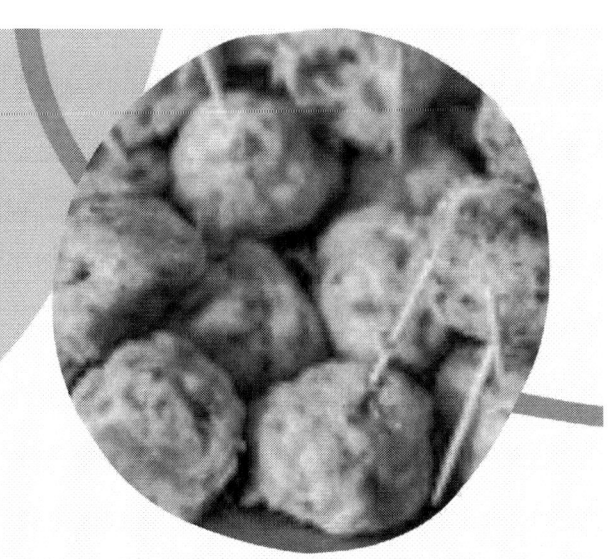

DIRECTIONS

1. Start by preheating the air fryer by setting the temperature to 350°F.
2. Take a glass bowl and add the ground chicken, green onions, cilantro, hoisin sauce, soy sauce, sriracha sauce, sesame oil, coconut, pepper, and salt. Mix well to combine.
3. Take the basket out of the air fryer and line it with foil. Use a small scooper and scoop out the mixture. Place the chicken in the basket lined with foil.
4. Return the basket to the fryer and cook for about 5 minutes. Flip over and cook for another 5 minutes.
5. Now increase the temperature to 400°F and cook for another 3 minutes until the chicken gets a nice brown color on top.
6. Serve with marinara sauce and spaghetti or dip of your choice.

Classic Chicken Thighs

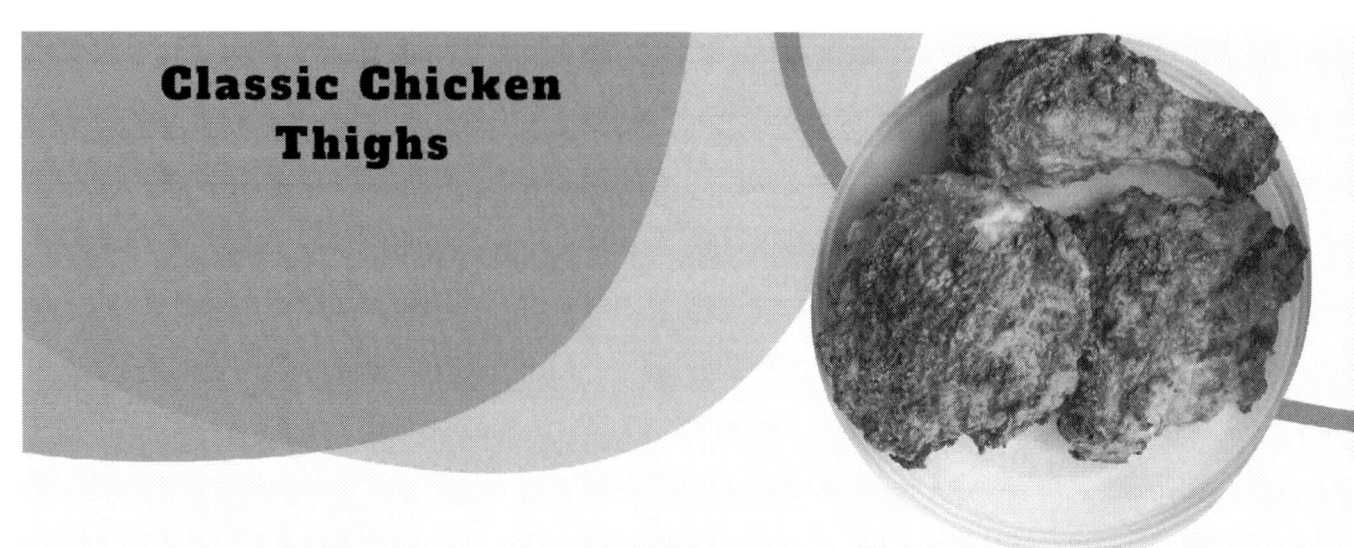

GENERAL INFO

Serving Size: 4
Servings per Recipe:
Calories: 213 calories per serving
Total Time: 30 minutes

INGREDIENTS

Chicken thighs (boneless) – 4
Olive oil (extra-virgin) – 2 teaspoons
Smoked paprika – 1 teaspoon
Garlic powder – ¾ teaspoon
Salt – ½ teaspoon
Black pepper (freshly ground) – ½ teaspoon

NUTRITION INFO

Fat – 14.2 g
Protein – 19.3 g
Carbohydrates – 0.9 g

Classic Chicken Thighs

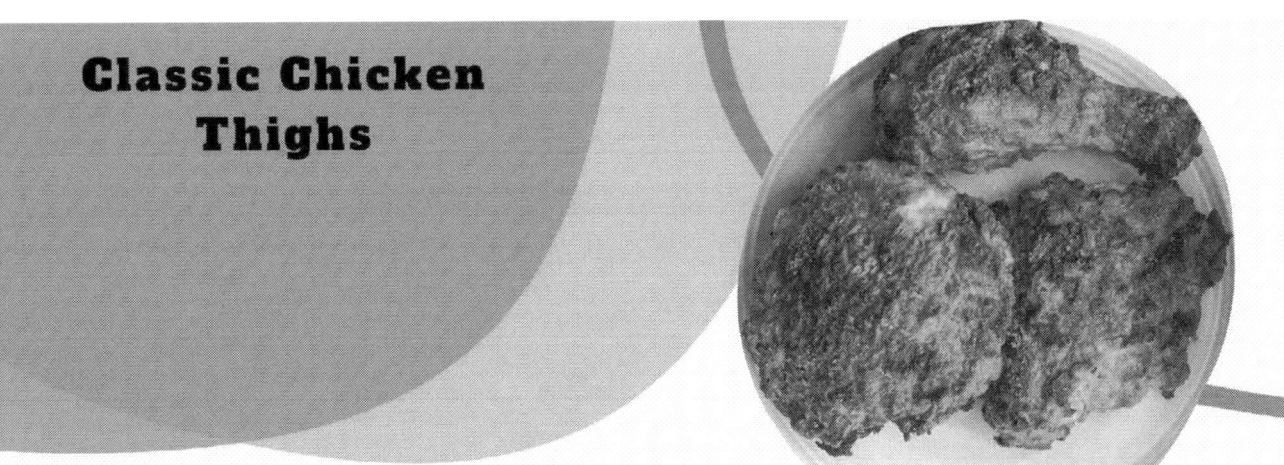

DIRECTIONS

1. Begin by preheating the air fryer by setting the temperature to 400°F.
2. In a medium glass mixing bowl, add the pepper, salt, garlic powder, and paprika. Mix well to combine.
3. Dry the chicken thighs using a kitchen paper towel. Use a brush to grease both sides of each thigh with extra-virgin olive oil.
4. Place the greased thighs in a shallow dish and sprinkle generously with the prepared spice mix. Flip over and sprinkle with the remaining spice mix. Make sure both sides of the thighs are evenly coated.
5. Take out the air fryer basket and place the seasoned thighs into the basket with the skin side facing up.
6. Transfer the chicken thighs into the air fryer and air-fry for about 18 minutes or until the thighs have a brown crust on top.
7. Take the chicken thighs out of the air fryer and place them on a serving platter.
8. Serve hot!

Crispy Low-Carb Fried Chicken

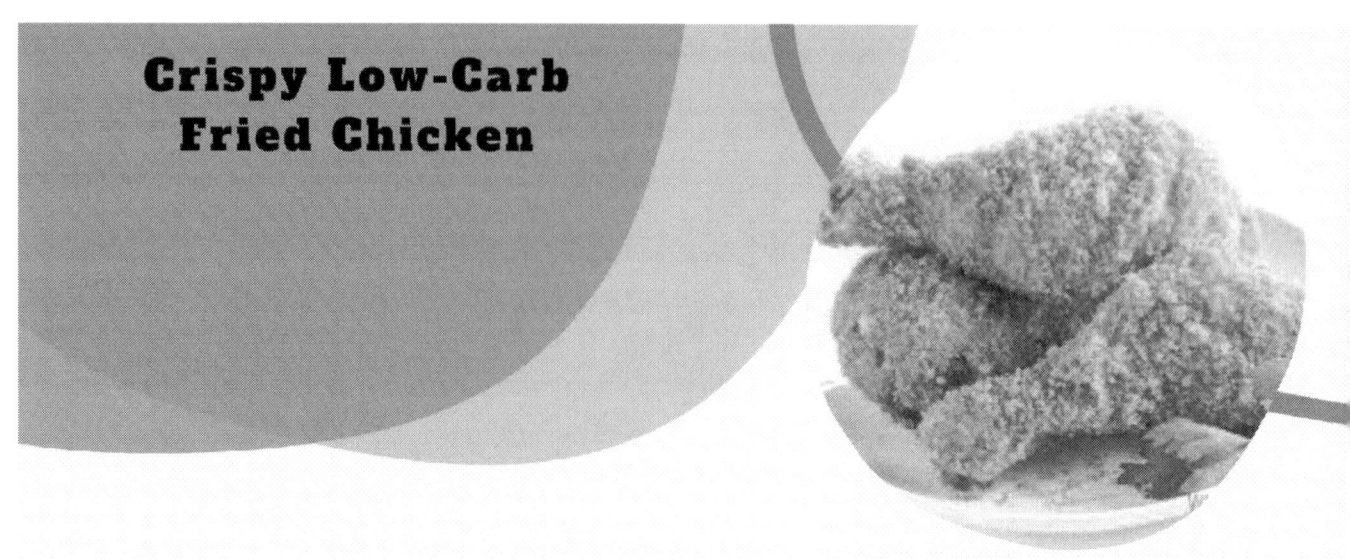

GENERAL INFO

Serving Size: 1
Servings per Recipe: 6
Calories: 378 calories per serving
Total Time: 57 minutes

INGREDIENTS

Plain kefir (whole-milk) – ½ cup
Hot sauce – 1 tablespoon
Chicken tenders – 1 ½ pounds
Pork rinds (crushed) – 2 packages
Parmesan cheese (finely grated) – 3 ounces
Garlic powder – 1 ½ teaspoons
Italian seasoning – ¾ teaspoon
Smoked sweet paprika – ½ teaspoon

NUTRITION INFO

Fat – 20.7 g
Protein – 47.4 g
Carbohydrates – 2.3 g

Crispy Low-Carb Fried Chicken

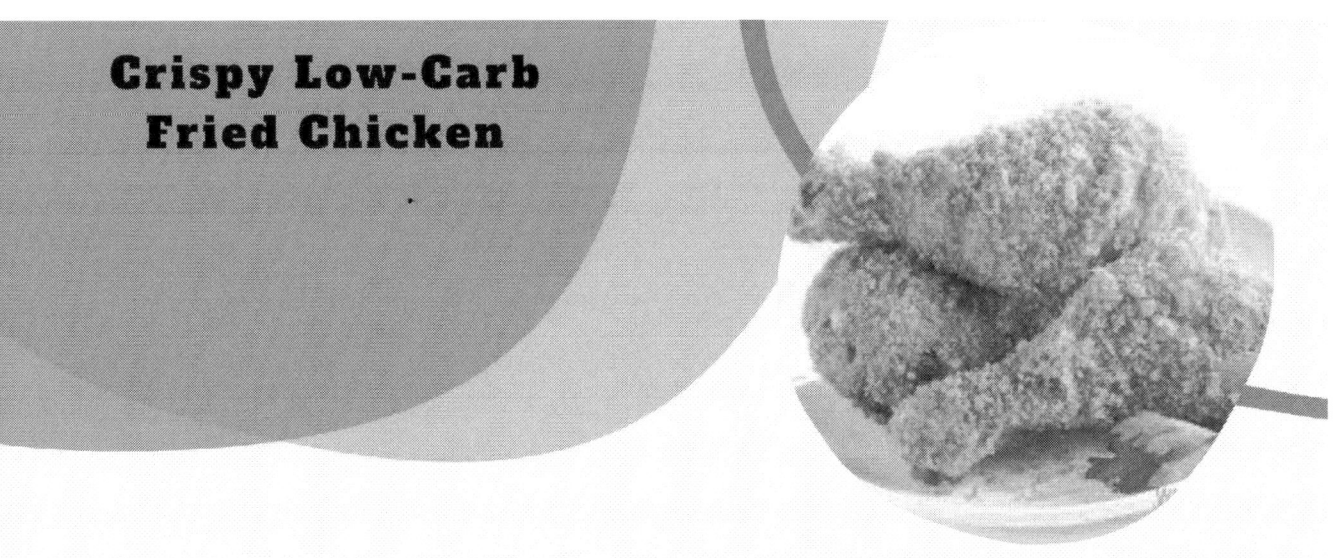

DIRECTIONS

1. Begin by taking a shallow bowl and adding the hot sauce and plain kefir. Mix well.
2. Now add the chicken tenders and let them sit in the marinade for about half an hour. (You can let them sit for an hour or more, depending on how much time you have available.)
3. Take another shallow dish and add the finely grated parmesan cheese, Italian seasoning, paprika, and garlic powder. Also add the crushed pork rind. Use a fork to mix well.
4. While the chicken is marinating, preheat the air fryer by setting the temperature to 390°F. Preheating should take about 3 minutes.
5. Use tongs to take the chicken out of the kefir marinade and dredge it evenly into the parmesan and pork rind mix.
6. Take out the air fryer basket and place the prepared chicken tenders into the same.
7. Transfer the basket to the air fryer and cook the chicken tenders for about 8 minutes. Flip over the chicken and cook for another 8 minutes. Cook for an additional 1 minute, if required.
8. Once done, transfer onto a serving platter and serve hot with chipotle dip or hot sauce.

Sesame Chicken Thighs

GENERAL INFO

Serving Size: 1
Servings per Recipe: 4
Calories: 485 calories per serving
Total Time: 55 minutes

INGREDIENTS

Sesame oil – 2 tablespoons
Soy sauce – 2 tablespoons
Honey – 1 tablespoon
Sriracha sauce – 1 tablespoon
Rice vinegar – 1 teaspoon
Chicken thighs – 2 pounds
Green onion (chopped) – 1
Sesame seeds (toasted) – 2 tablespoons

NUTRITION INFO

Fat – 32.6 g
Protein – 39.5 g
Carbohydrates – 6.6 g

Sesame Chicken Thighs

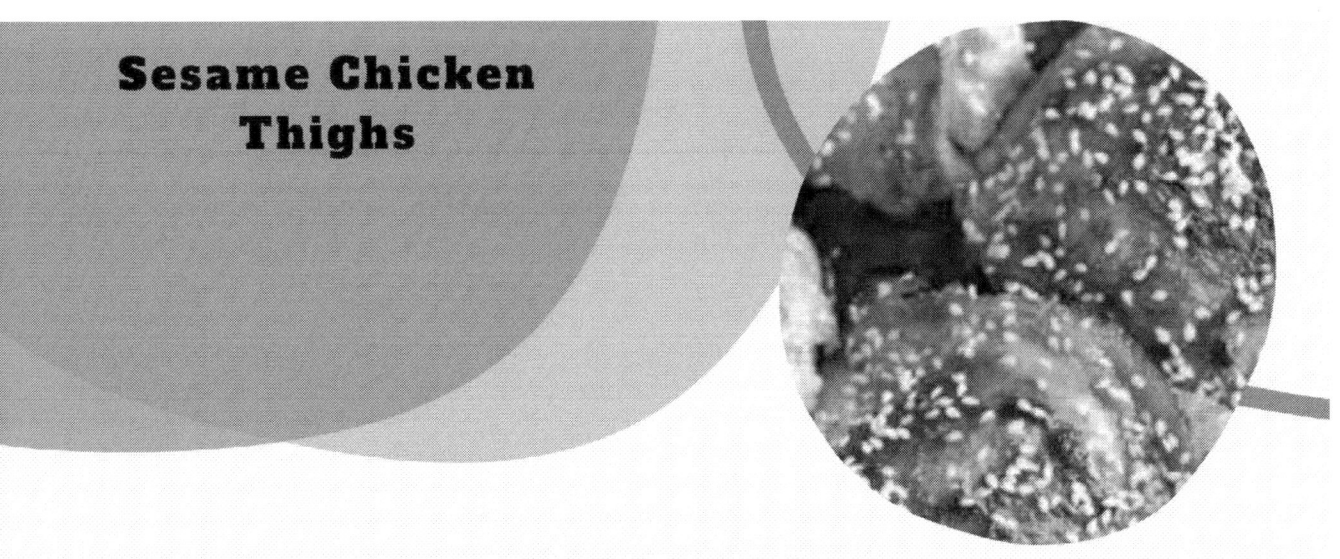

DIRECTIONS

1. Start by combining the soy sauce, sesame oil, sriracha, vinegar, and honey in a mixing bowl.
2. Add the chicken thighs to the soy sauce mixture and cover with a cling film. Let it sit in the refrigerator for about 30 minutes.
3. While the chicken is marinating, preheat the air fryer by setting the temperature to 400°F.
4. Take the chicken out of the fridge and set aside.
5. Take out the air fryer basket and place the chicken thigh on the same. (Fry in batches if required.) Discard the marinade.
6. Transfer the basket back into the air fryer and cook for about 5 minutes.
7. Open the basket, flip the chicken thigh over, and cook for another 10 minutes.
8. Once done, transfer the air-fried chicken onto a serving platter and let it stand for about 5 minutes.
9. Finish by garnishing with chopped sesame seeds and green onion. Serve hot with the dip of your choice!

Turkey Breast

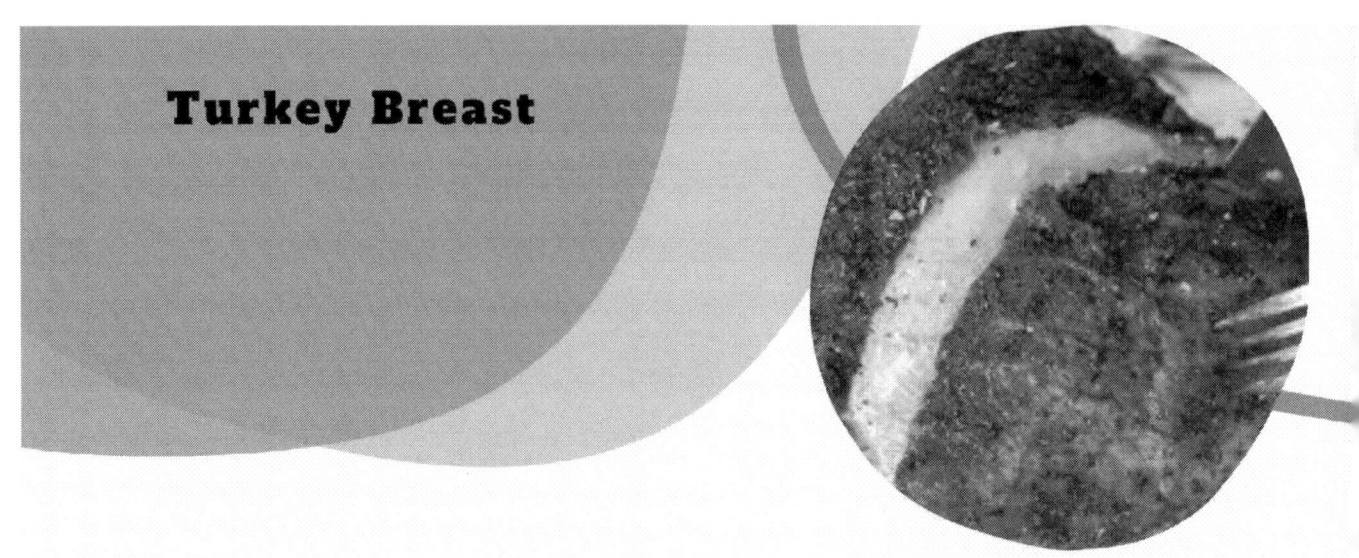

GENERAL INFO

Serving Size: 1
Servings per Recipe: 6
Calories: 263 calories per serving
Total Time: 1 hour

INGREDIENTS

Fresh rosemary (finely chopped) – 1 tablespoon
Fresh chives (finely chopped) – 1 teaspoon
Fresh garlic (finely minced) – 1 teaspoon
Salt – ½ teaspoon
Black pepper (freshly ground) – ¼ teaspoon
Unsalted butter – 2 tablespoons
Split turkey breast (skin-on and bone-in) – 2 ¾ pounds
Chives (chopped) – for garnishing

NUTRITION INFO

Fat – 10.1 g
Protein – 40.2 g
Carbohydrates – 0.3 g

Turkey Breast

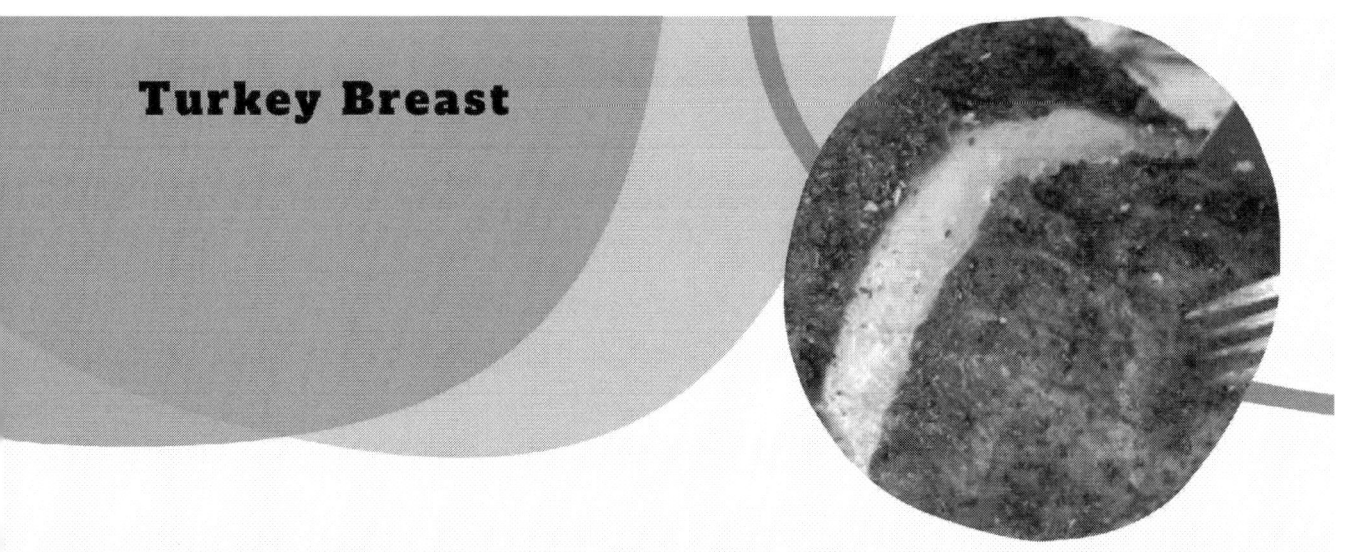

DIRECTIONS

1. Start by preheating the air fryer by setting the temperature to 350°F.
2. Take a chopping board and place the chives, rosemary, salt, pepper, and garlic on it. Also, add 2 tablespoons of butter to the chopping board. Mince all the ingredients together. Your herb butter is ready.
3. Use a kitchen towel to pat the turkey breast dry.
4. Now evenly spread the herb butter on both sides of the turkey. Make sure to generously apply the herb butter beneath the turkey skin.
5. Take out the basket from the air fryer and place the herbed turkey breasts in the center. Make sure the skin side of the turkey faces down.
6. Let the turkey cook for about 20 minutes. Flip over and cook for another 18 minutes.
7. Once done, transfer onto a platter and cover with heavy aluminum foil. Let the turkey breasts rest for about 10 minutes before slicing.
8. Serve hot with a sprinkle of fresh chives.

An Appeal from the Publisher

Hello wonderful reader!

We hope you are enjoying this book.

We wanted to let you know that you have made an impact on many lives by purchasing this book.

Just to give you a brief introduction: We are a small publishing company with a team of 8 writers and 2 editors.

Most of our employees come from financially weaker section and our company is the only means they support their families. This is our way of giving back to the society.

We don't have the giant advertising budgets that many other publishers and businesses do online.

So, one way that you can really support our mission and our business is by leaving us a review on this book.

For a small company like us, getting reviews (especially on Amazon) means we can submit our books for advertising.

This means we can actually sell a few copies from time to time and make a bigger impact on the society as a whole. So, every review means a lot to us.

We can't THANK YOU enough for this!

beef, pork, and lamb
RECIPES

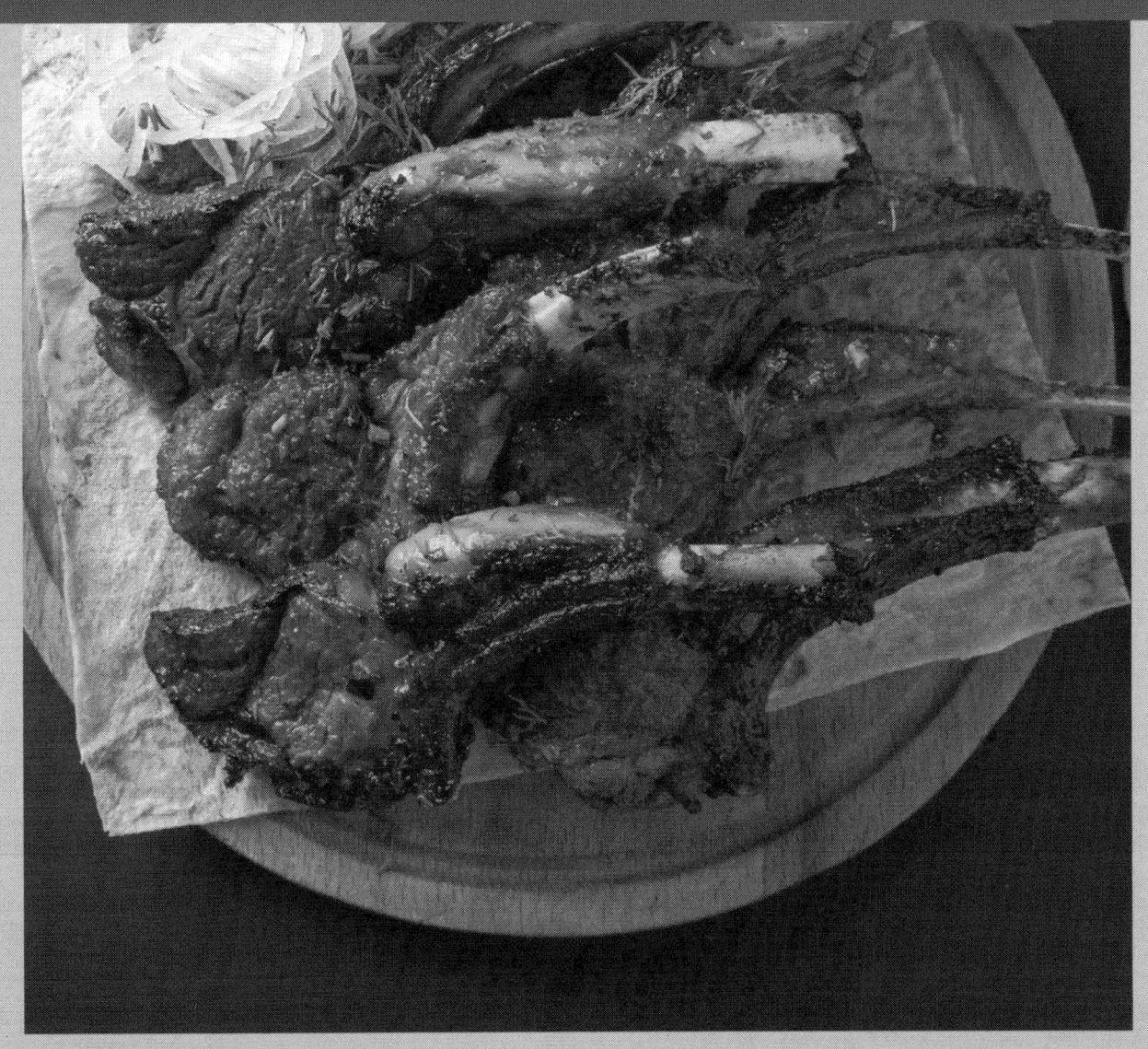

Air-Fried Beef Meatloaf

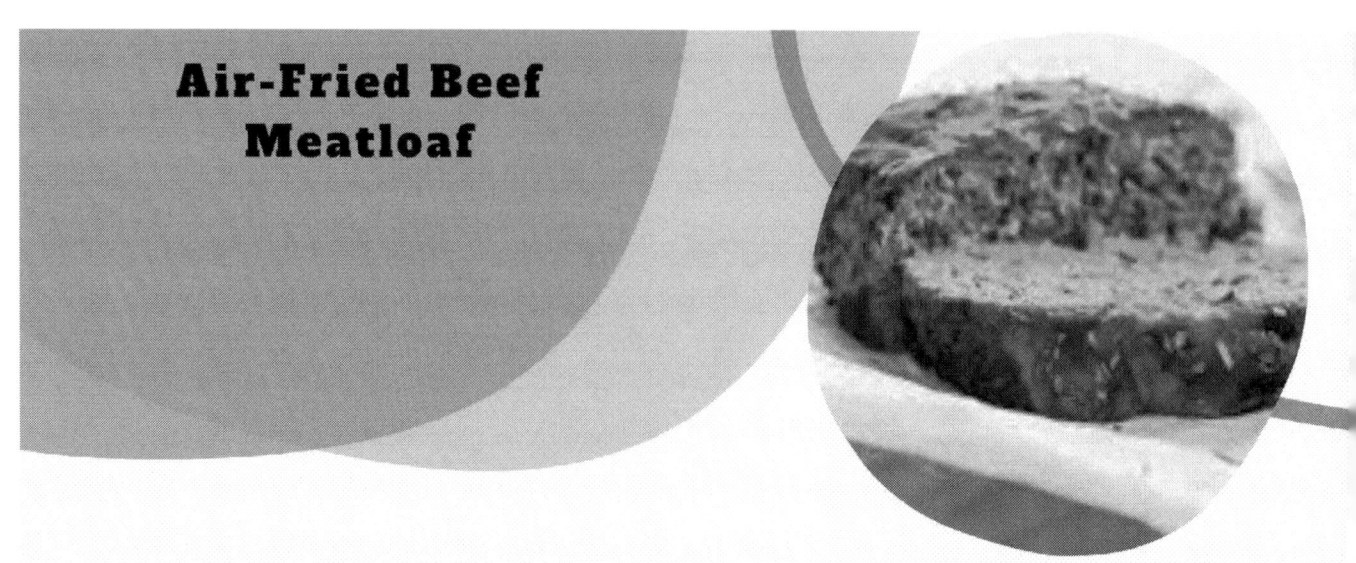

GENERAL INFO

Serving Size: 1
Servings per Recipe: 4
Calories: 260 calories per serving
Total Time: 28 minutes

INGREDIENTS

Lean beef (ground) – 1 pound
Eggs – 2
Onion (diced) – 1 cup
Cilantro (chopped) – ¼ cup
Ginger (minced) – 1 tablespoon
Garlic (minced) – 1 tablespoon
Garam masala – 2 teaspoon
Salt – 1 teaspoon
Turmeric – 1 teaspoon
Cayenne – 1 teaspoon
Cinnamon (ground) – ½ teaspoon
Cardamom (ground) – ⅛ teaspoon

NUTRITION INFO

Fat – 13 g
Protein – 26 g
Carbohydrates – 6 g

Air-Fried Beef Meatloaf

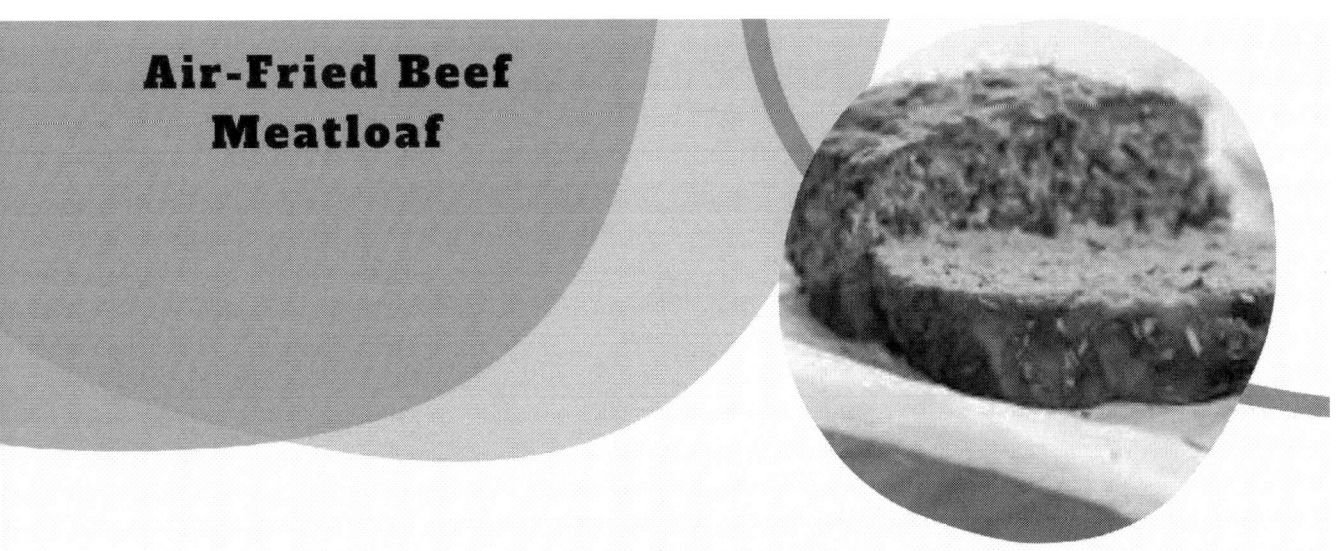

DIRECTIONS

1. Start by taking a large bowl and add the ground lean eggs, cilantro, beef, ginger, garlic, onion, salt, garam masala, turmeric, cardamom, cinnamon, and cayenne. Use your hands to mix well until combined.
2. Take an 8-inch tin pan and transfer the beef mixture into the same.
3. Place the tin into the air fryer basket and cook for 15 minutes at 360°F.
4. Once done, remove the pan from the air fryer and set aside.
5. Drain any excess liquid and transfer the meatloaf onto a flat wooden surface.
6. Slice the loaf into 4 equal pieces. Serve hot

Air-Fried Bun Thit Nuong

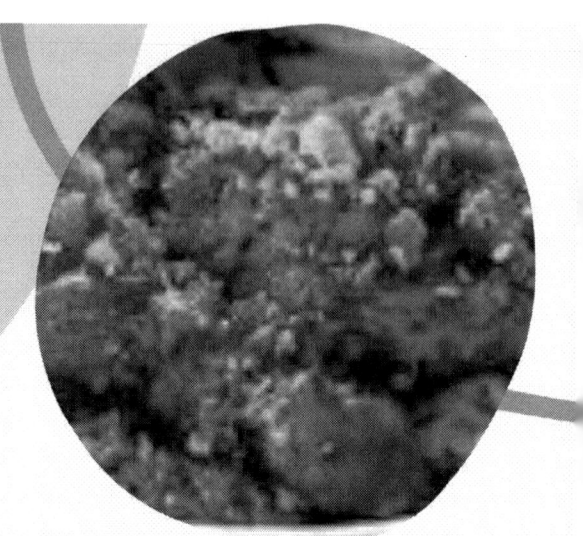

GENERAL INFO

Serving Size: 1
Servings per Recipe: 4
Calories: 231 calories per serving
Total Time: 50 minutes

INGREDIENTS

Onions (chopped) – ¼ cup
Olive oil – 2 tablespoons
Sugar – 2 tablespoons
Dark soy sauce – 2 teaspoons
Garlic (minced) – 1 tablespoon
Fish sauce – 1 tablespoon
Lemongrass paste (minced) – 1 tablespoon
Black pepper (freshly ground) – ½ teaspoon
Pork shoulder (thinly sliced) – 1 pound

For garnishing
Roasted peanuts (crushed) – ¼ cup
Cilantro (chopped) – 2 tablespoons

NUTRITION INFO

Fat – 16 g
Protein – 16 g
Carbohydrates – 4 g

Air-Fried Bun Thit Nuong

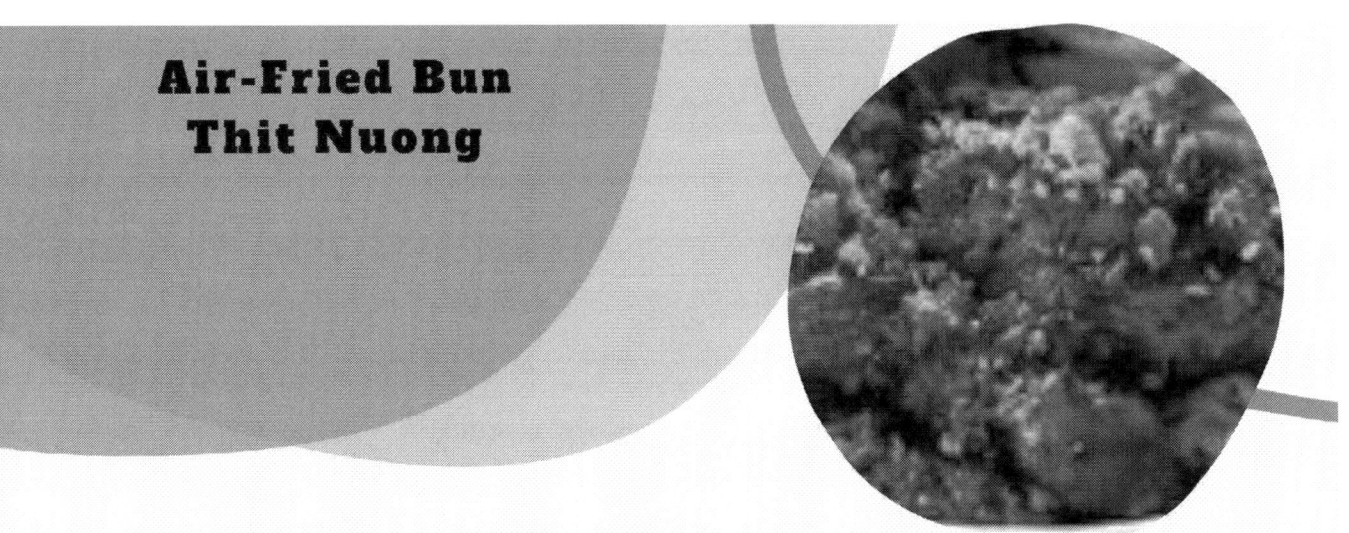

DIRECTIONS

1. Take a large bowl and add the onions, soy sauce, garlic, sugar, oil, lemongrass, pepper, and fish sauce. Your marinade is ready.
2. Place the pork shoulder onto a chopping board and cut it into 4 x ½-inch pieces.
3. Toss the pork shoulder strips into the marinade. Let it sit for about half an hour.
4. Place the marinated pork strips into the air fryer basket and cook for about 5 minutes at 400°F. Flip over and cook for another 5 minutes.
5. Once done, transfer the pork onto a serving tray.
6. Finish by sprinkling with roasted peanuts and cilantro.

Beef Satay in an Air Fryer

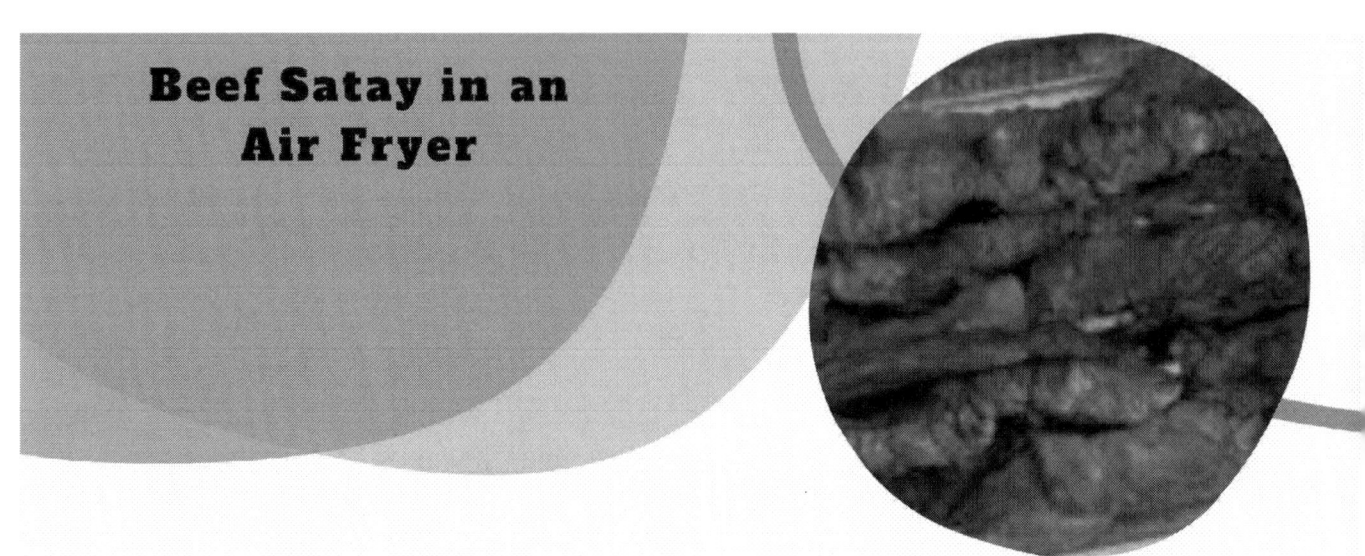

GENERAL INFO

Serving Size: 1
Servings per Recipe: 2
Calories: 582 calories per serving
Total Time: 43 minutes

INGREDIENTS

Flank steak (cut in long strips) – 1 pound
Oil – 2 tablespoons
Fish sauce – 1 tablespoon
Soy sauce – 1 tablespoon
Ginger (minced) – 1 tablespoon
Garlic (minced) – 1 tablespoon
Sugar – 1 tablespoon
Sriracha sauce – 1 teaspoon
Coriander powder – 1 teaspoon
Cilantro (chopped) – ½ cup
Roasted peanuts (chopped) – ¼ cup

NUTRITION INFO

Fat – 34 g
Protein – 56 g
Carbohydrates – 12 g

Beef Satay in an Air Fryer

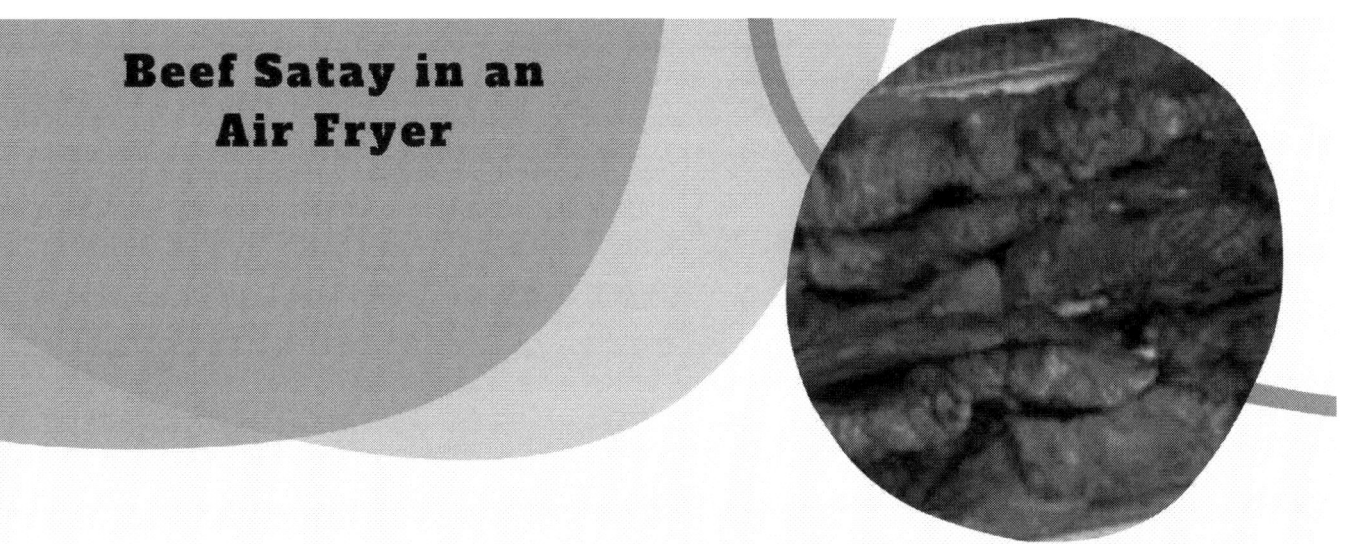

DIRECTIONS

1. Begin by placing the beef strips into a large mixing bowl.
2. Add the fish sauce, oil, ginger, soy sauce, garlic, sriracha, sugar, ¼ cup of cilantro, and coriander powder. Mix well until the beef strips are evenly coated.
3. Cover the bowl with cling film and let the steak strips marinate for almost 30 minutes in the refrigerator.
4. Once done, place the coated steak strips into the air fryer basket. Discard the marinade.
5. Turn on the air fryer and cook for 4 minutes at 400°F. Flip over and cook for another 4 minutes.
6. Transfer the cooked steak strips onto a serving platter and top with the remaining cilantro and roasted peanuts.
7. Serve with peanut sauce or any other dip of your choice.

Cumin and Sichuan Lamb

GENERAL INFO

Serving Size: 1
Servings per Recipe: 4
Calories: 170 calories per serving
Total Time: 25 minutes

INGREDIENTS

For lamb
Cumin – 2 tablespoons
Sichuan peppers – 1 teaspoon
Lamb shoulder (cut in 2-inch pieces) – 1 pound
Vegetable oil – 2 tablespoons
Light soy sauce – 1 tablespoon
Garlic (minced) – 1 tablespoons
Red chili peppers – 2
Salt – 1 teaspoon
Sugar – ¼ teaspoon

For garnishing
Scallions (chopped) – 2
Cilantro (chopped) – 1 handful

NUTRITION INFO

Fat – 11 g
Protein – 15 g
Carbohydrates – 2 g

Cumin and Sichuan Lamb

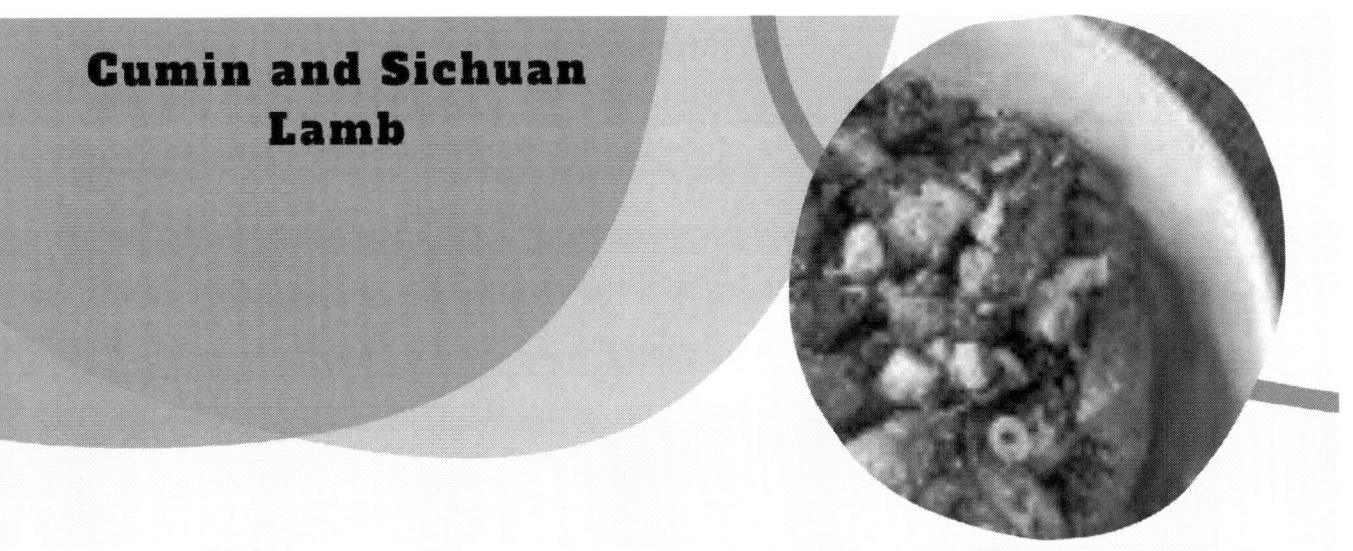

DIRECTIONS

1. Start by preparing the spice mix to marinate the lamb. For this, you need to take a dry non-stick pan and add the cumin and Sichuan pepper. Roast them until they become fragrant.
2. Empty the cumin and pepper into a mortar and pestle. Allow them to cool. Once cooled, grind them into a coarse powder.
3. Poke holes into the lamb shoulder and place it in a shallow dish. Sprinkle the prepared spice mix on top and use your hand to massage the meat.
4. Add the oil, light soy sauce, red chili peppers, garlic, sugar, cayenne pepper, and sugar. Mix and massage well into the pork shoulder.
5. Turn on the air fryer and place the marinated pork into the basket.
6. Cook the pork for 10 minutes at 360°F.
7. Transfer the lamb shoulder onto a serving platter.
8. Finish by garnishing with chopped cilantro and scallions. Serve hot!

Flank Steak Topped with Zhoug

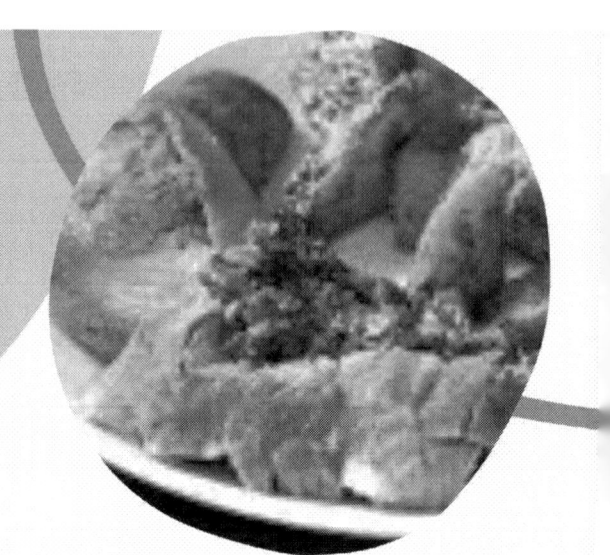

GENERAL INFO

Serving Size: 1
Servings per Recipe: 4
Calories: 410 calories per serving
Total Time: 28 minutes

NUTRITION INFO

Fat – 23 g
Protein – 37 g
Carbohydrates – 10 g

INGREDIENTS

For marinade
Dark beer – ½ cup
Lemon juice – 1/4 cups
Olive oil – 2 tablespoons
Sriracha sauce – 2 tablespoons
Brown sugar – 2 tablespoons
Ground cumin – 2 teaspoons
Smoked paprika – 2 teaspoons
Salt – 1 tablespoon
Ground black pepper – 1 teaspoon
Garlic (minced) – 3 cloves
Flank steak – 1.5 pounds

For zhoug
Cilantro leaves – 1 cup
Garlic – 2 cloves
Jalapeno (coarsely chopped) – 2
Ground cumin – ½ teaspoon
Ground coriander – ¼ teaspoon
Salt – ¼ teaspoon
Olive oil – 4 tablespoons

Flank Steak Topped with Zhoug

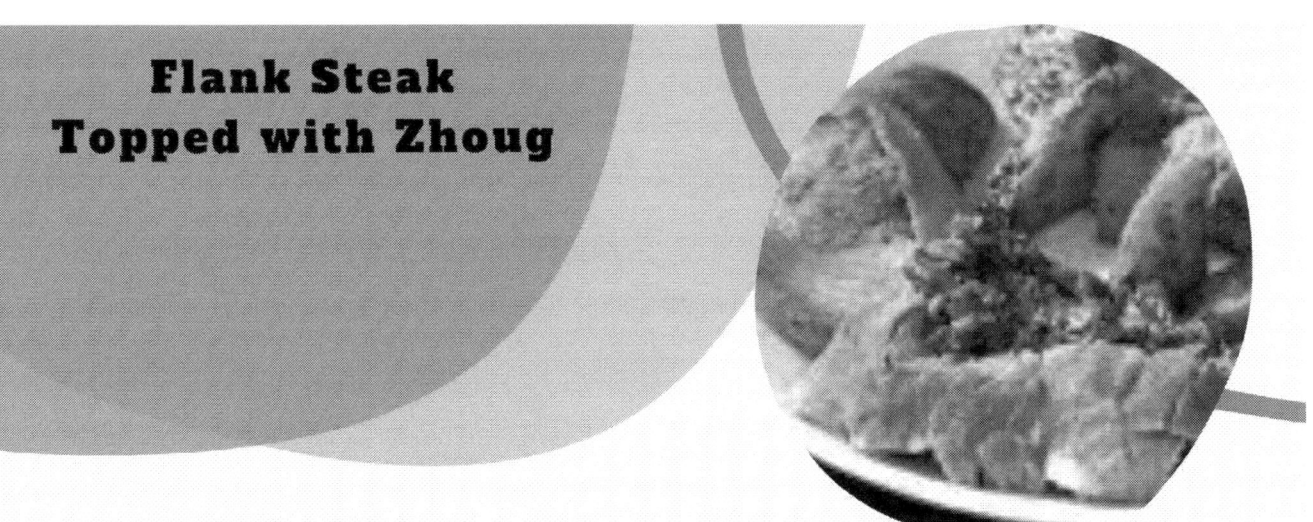

DIRECTIONS

1. Start by trimming the flank steak and cut it into 3 equal pieces.
2. Preparing the marinade: Take a small mixing bowl and add the beer, olive oil, lemon juice, cumin, sriracha, salt, smoked paprika, garlic, and black pepper. Whisk well to combine.
3. Take a large zip-lock bag and place the steak inside the same. Pour the marinade over the steak and seal the bag. Shake until both sides are well-coated.
4. Place the zip-lock bag into the refrigerator for about 1 hour and let the steak marinate.
5. While the steak is marinating, prepare the zhoug. Take a food processor and add the cilantro, jalapeno, garlic, coriander, salt, and cumin. Process until well-combined and finely chopped.
6. Slowly add about 4 tablespoons of olive oil and pulse until well-combined. The zhoug is ready.
7. Transfer the prepared zhoug into a container and place it in the refrigerator for 30 minutes.
8. While the zhoug is cooling, take the steak out of the refrigerator. Let it sit for about 5 minutes.
9. Now remove the steak from the zip-lock bag and place it in the air fryer basket. Discard the rest of the marinade. Cook the steak for 10 minutes at 400°F.
10. Remove the steak from the air fryer and place it on a wooden block. Let it sit for about 5 minutes before slicing.
11. Cut the steak into ½-inch-thick slices and transfer it onto a serving platter. Serve hot!

German-Style Rouladen

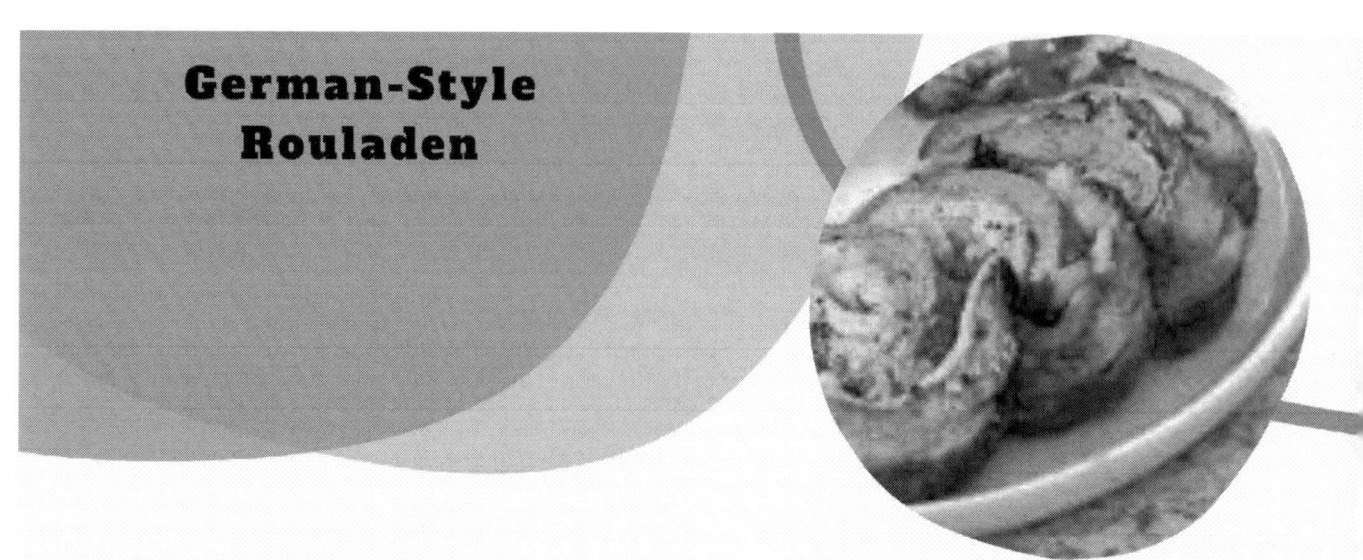

GENERAL INFO

Serving Size: 1
Servings per Recipe: 4
Calories: 443 calories per serving
Total Time: 28 minutes

INGREDIENTS

Sauce
Oil – 3 tablespoons
Onion (sliced) – 2 cups
Sour cream – ½ cup
Tomato paste – 1 tablespoon
Dill pickles (chopped) – ¼ cup
Parsley (chopped) – 1 teaspoon

Steak
Flank steak – 1 pound
Dijon mustard – ¼ cup
Black pepper (freshly ground) – 1 teaspoon
Bacon – 4
Parsley (chopped) – ¼ cup

NUTRITION INFO

Fat – 39 g
Protein – 21 g
Carbohydrates – 10 g

German-Style Rouladen

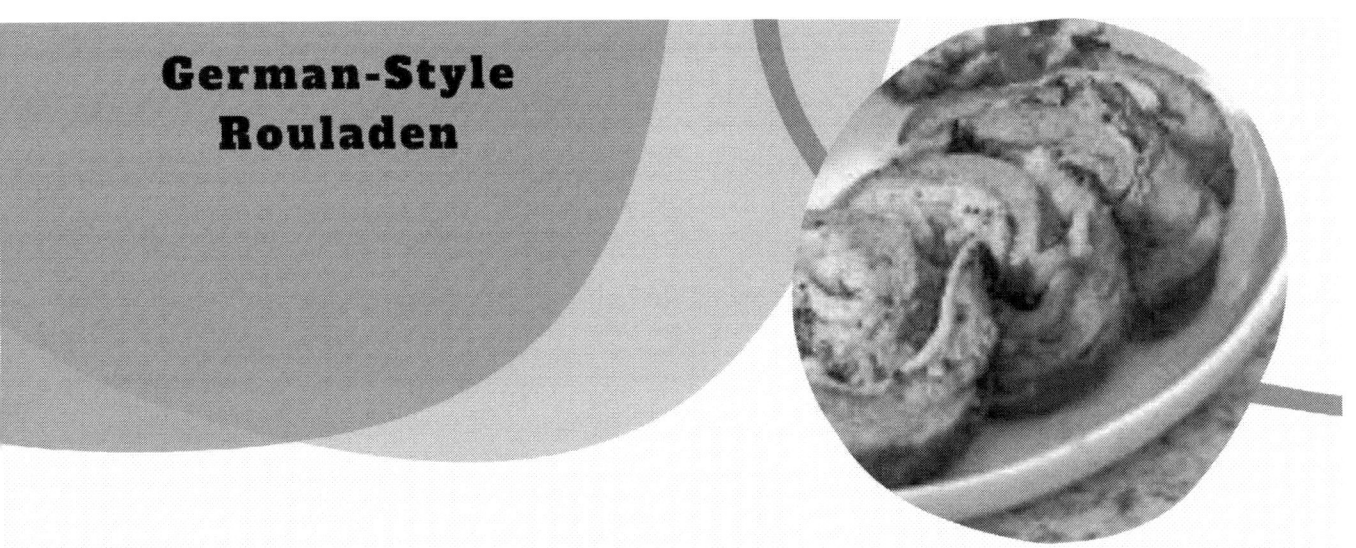

DIRECTIONS

1. Start by taking a mixing bowl and add the sliced onion, ½ teaspoon of pepper, and ½ teaspoon of salt. Mix well.
2. Turn on the air fryer and place the coated seasoned onions in it. Cook for 5 minutes at 400°F.
3. Once done, set aside half of the cooked onions for later use. Place the remaining half of cooked onions into a bowl and also add the tomato paste, sour cream, 2 teaspoons parsley, and chopped dill pickles. Stir in about 2 tablespoons of water to obtain a runny consistency. Your sauce is ready.
4. To prepare the steak, place the meat on a plate and evenly spread Dijon mustard on the top. Place the cooked onions, bacon slices, and chopped parsley over the meat.
5. Tightly roll up the flank steak and secure with a toothpick. Use a knife to cut the steak roll into 2 equal halves.
6. Place the prepared steak rolls into the air fryer basket and cook for about 10 minutes at 400°F.
7. Transfer the steak onto a serving platter and serve hot with the prepared sauce.

Lamb Sirloin Steaks in an Air Fryer

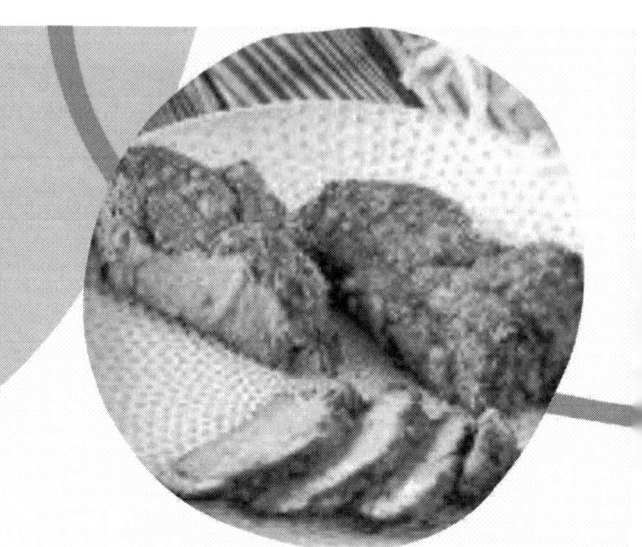

GENERAL INFO

Serving Size: 1
Servings per Recipe: 4
Calories: 182 calories per serving
Total Time: 55 minutes

INGREDIENTS

Onion – ½
Ginger – 4 slices
Garlic – 5 cloves
Garam masala – 1 teaspoon
Ground fennel – 1 teaspoon
Ground cinnamon – 1 teaspoon
Ground cardamom – ½ teaspoon
Cayenne pepper – 1 teaspoon
Salt – 1 teaspoon
Lamb sirloin steaks (boneless) – 1 pound

NUTRITION INFO

Fat – 7 g
Protein – 24 g
Carbohydrates – 3 g

Lamb Sirloin Steaks in an Air Fryer

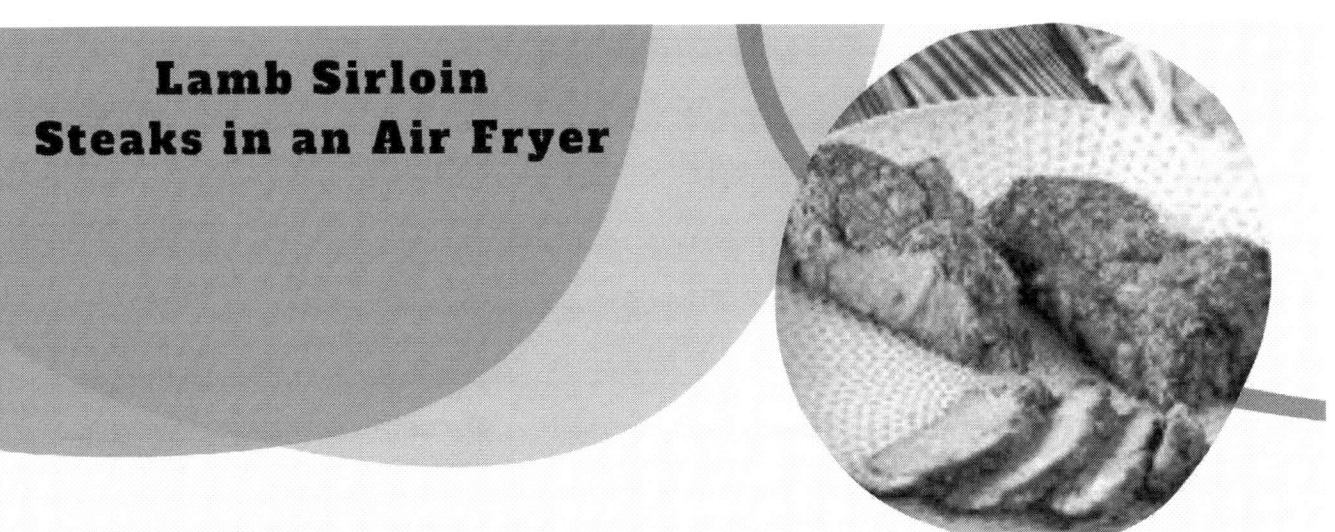

DIRECTIONS

1. Start by adding onion, ginger, garlic, garam masala, ground fennel, ground cinnamon, ground cardamom, cayenne pepper, and salt to a food processor.
2. Pulse until the onion is finely chopped and well-blended with the other ingredients. This will take about 4 minutes.
3. Take a large mixing bowl and place the lamb chops inside the same. Make small cuts in the steaks using a knife. (This will help in infusing flavor into the meat.)
4. Add the prepared spice mix and combine well. Let the sirloin steaks marinate in the spice mix for almost 30 minutes in the refrigerator.
5. Once the lamb is done marinating, place the steaks into the air fryer basket and cook for 8 minutes at 330°F. Flip over and cook for 7 more minutes.
6. Transfer the steak onto a wooden chopping block and cut into slices.
7. Serve hot!

Pork Chops in an Air Fryer

GENERAL INFO

Serving Size: 1
Servings per Recipe: 2
Calories: 201 calories per serving
Total Time: 25 minutes

NUTRITION INFO

Fat – 21 g
Protein – 4 g
Carbohydrates – 1 g

INGREDIENTS

Olive oil – 2 tablespoons
Fresh rosemary (chopped) – 2 teaspoons
Fresh sage (chopped finely) – 1 teaspoon
Fennel seeds (crushed lightly) – 1 teaspoon
Red pepper flakes – ½ teaspoon
Salt – 1 teaspoon
Black pepper (freshly ground) – 1 teaspoon
Garlic (minced) – 2 cloves
Lemon zest – 1
Olive oil – 1 tablespoon
Bone-in pork chops (center cut) – 16 ounces, 1 inch thick
Kosher salt – as per taste
Pepper (freshly ground) – as per taste

Pork Chops in an Air Fryer

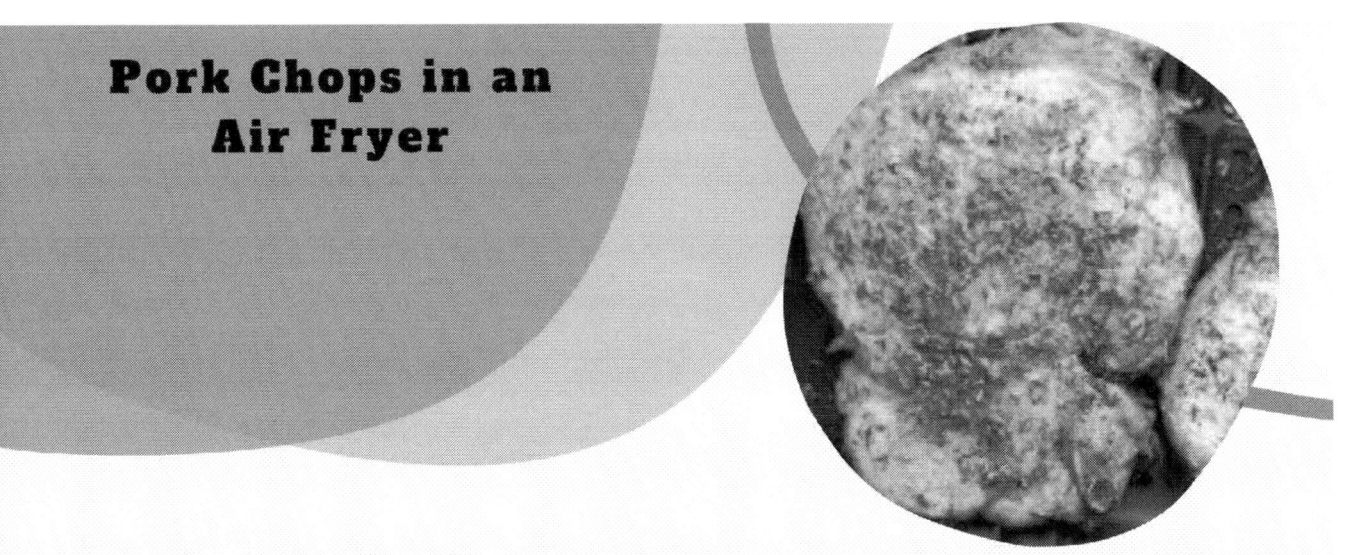

DIRECTIONS

1. Start by combining the rosemary, fennel seeds, sage, crushed red pepper, pepper, garlic, salt, 1 tablespoon of olive oil, and lemon zest. Mix until all ingredients are well-combined.
2. Place the pork chops onto a flat surface and cut them into 1-inch slices.
3. Place the pork chops in a shallow dish and coat them evenly with the prepared herb mix.
4. Place the prepared pork chops into the air fryer basket for about 15 minutes at 380°F.
5. Once done, transfer the pork chops onto a serving a platter.
6. Serve hot!

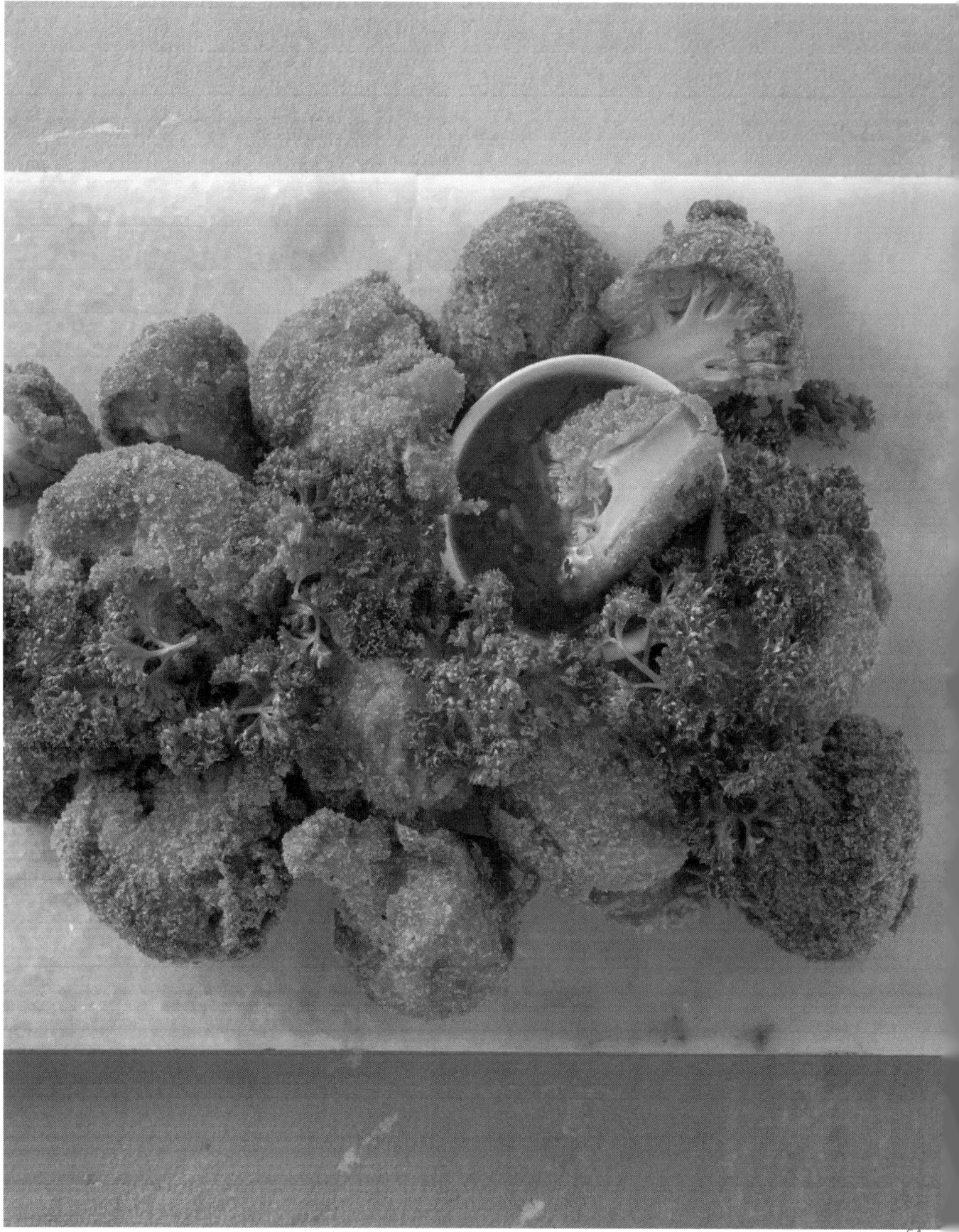

vegetarian
RECIPES

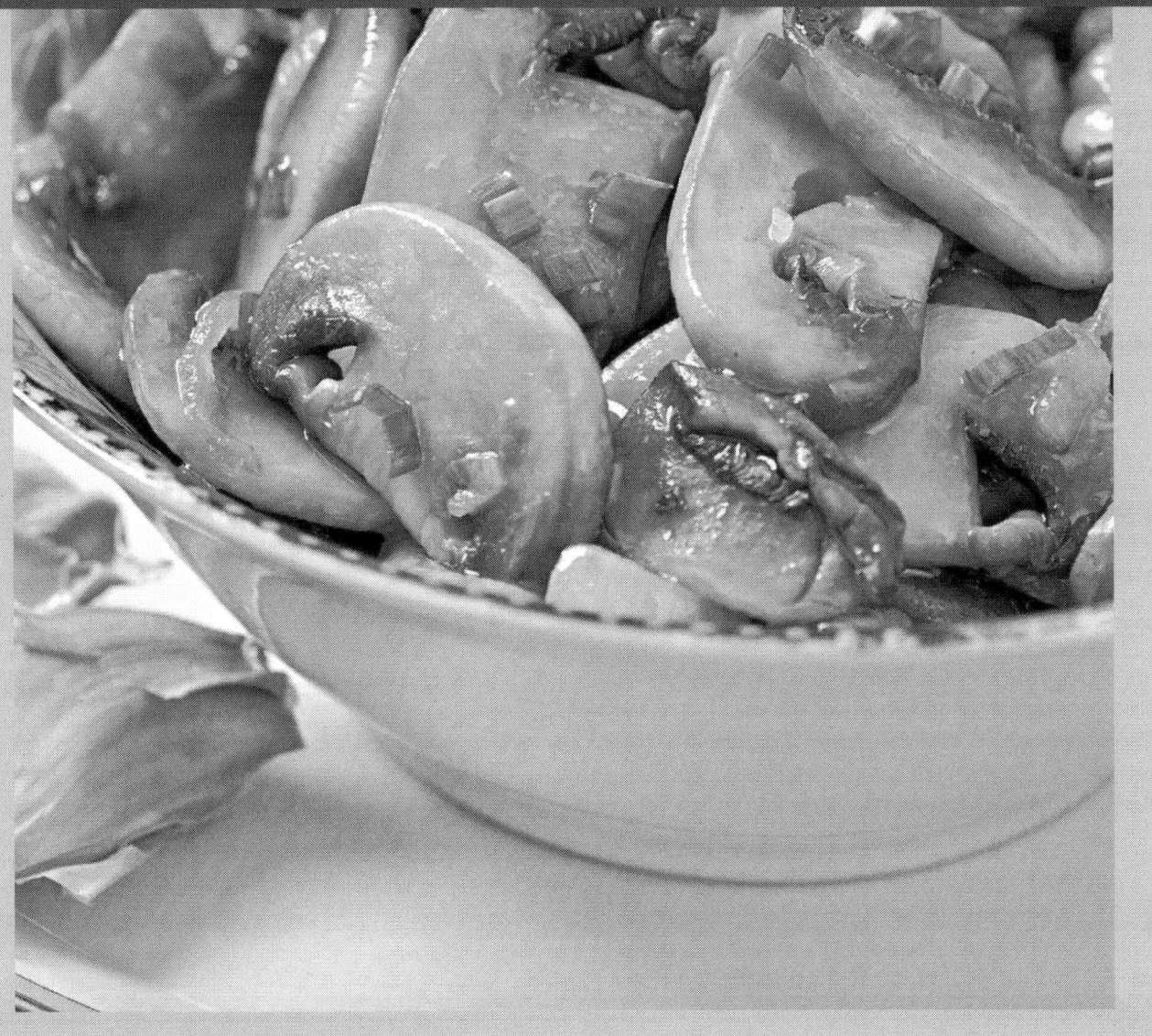

Air-Fried Eggplant Pizza

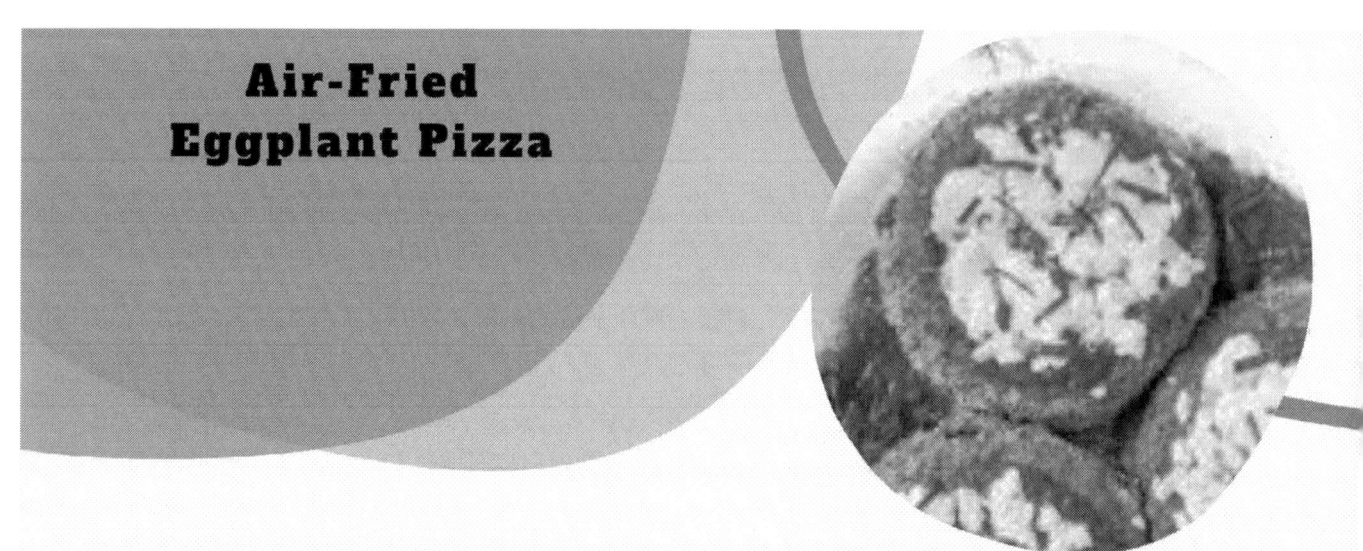

GENERAL INFO

Serving Size: 1
Servings per Recipe: 8
Calories: 80 calories per serving
Total Time: 25 minutes

INGREDIENTS

Eggplant (sliced) – 1
Olive oil – 2 tablespoons
Tomato sauce – ½ cup
Mozzarella cheese – ¾ cup
Olive oil spray

NUTRITION INFO

Fat – 6 g
Protein – 3 g
Carbohydrates – 4 g

Air-Fried Eggplant Pizza

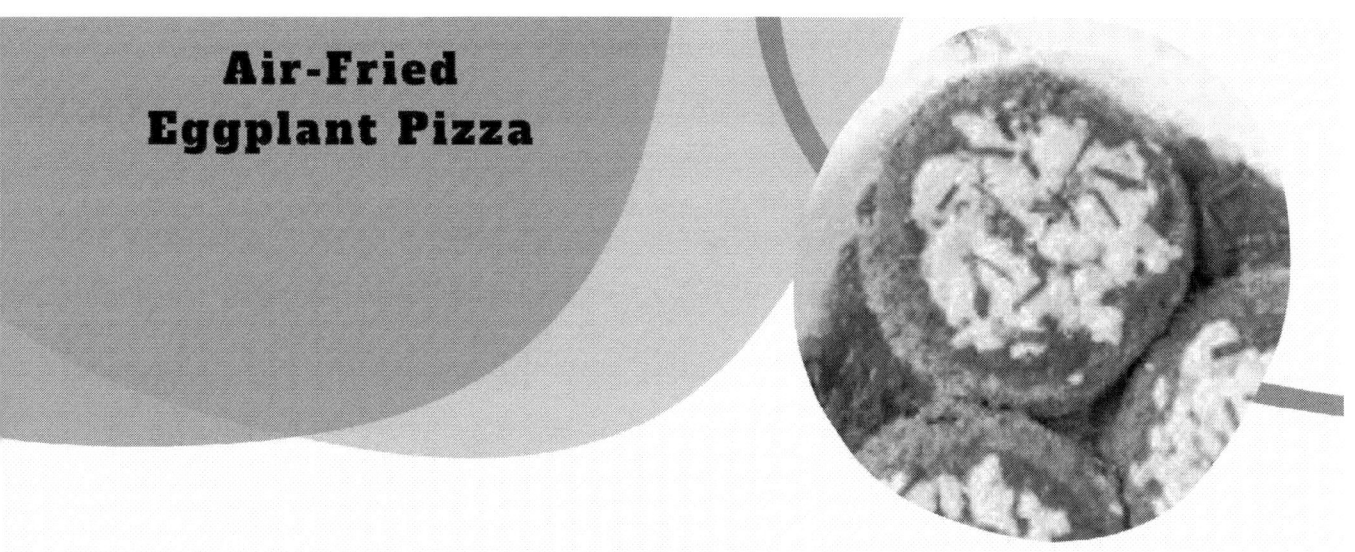

DIRECTIONS

1. Begin by prepping the air fryer basket by spraying it with olive oil spray.
2. Turn on the air fryer and let it preheat at 400°F.
3. While the air fryer is preheating, prepare the eggplant slices. For this, brush all the slices generously with olive oil.
4. Arrange the eggplant slices into the preheated air fryer basket in a single layer. Cook for 10 minutes.
5. Remove the basket and flip over the slices. Cook for another 3 minutes. (Cook in batches if necessary.)
6. Transfer the cooked eggplant slices over a flat wooden surface. Spread tomato sauce evenly over all the eggplant slices.
7. Top these slices with cheese and return them to the air fryer basket. Cook for about 3 minutes or until the cheese begins to melt.
8. Serve hot!

Chermoula Air-Fried Beets

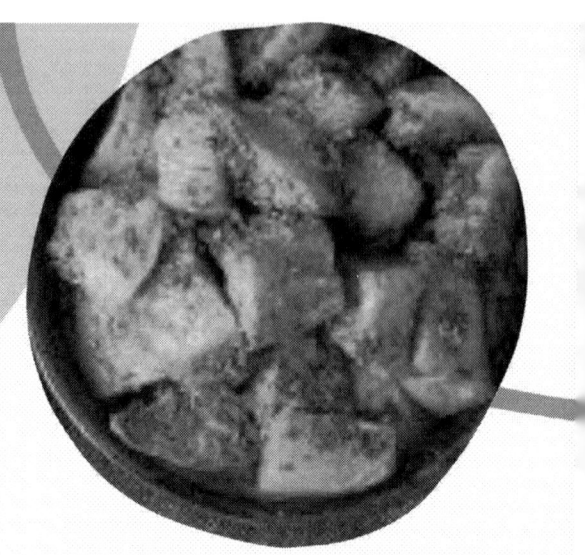

GENERAL INFO

Serving Size: 1
Servings per Recipe: 4
Calories: 283 calories per serving
Total Time: 35

INGREDIENTS

Cilantro leaves – 1 cup
Parsley leaves – ½ cup
Garlic – 6 cloves
Smoked paprika – 2 teaspoons
Cumin powder – 2 teaspoons
Coriander powder – 1 teaspoon
Cayenne – ½ teaspoon
Saffron strands – a pinch
Olive oil – ½ cup
Kosher salt – as per taste
Beets – 3 medium, trimmed, peeled and cut into 1-inch chunks
Cilantro (chopped) – 2 tablespoons
Parsley (chopped) – 2 tablespoons
Lemon juice – 1 teaspoon

NUTRITION INFO

Fat – 27 g
Protein – 2 g
Carbohydrates – 9 g

Chermoula Air-Fried Beets

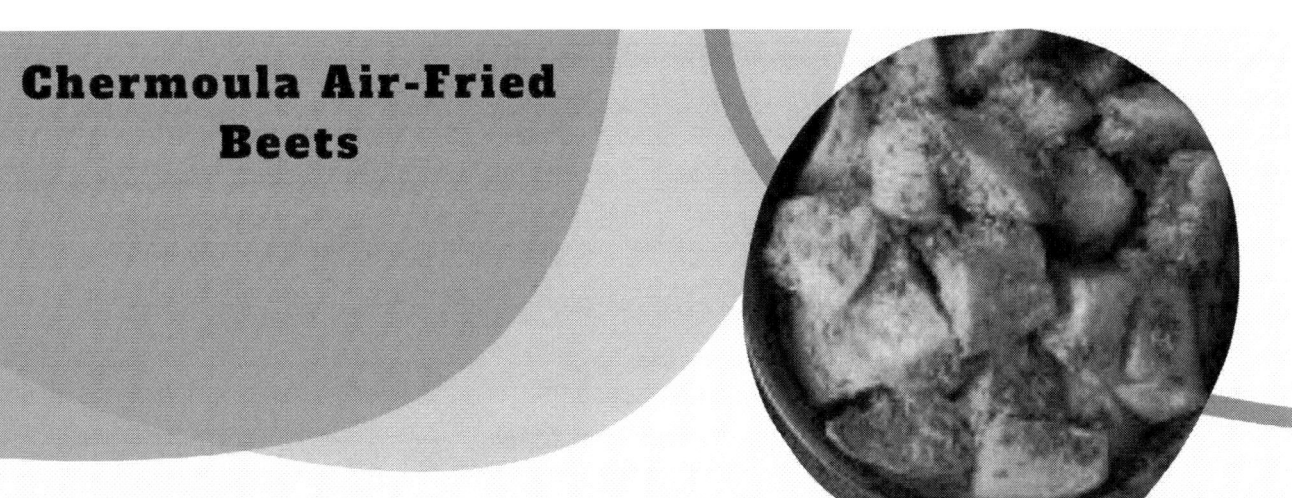

DIRECTIONS

1. Start by trimming and peeling the beets. Cut them into chunks measuring about 1 inch each.
2. Add the cilantro leaves, parsley leaves, smoked paprika, garlic, coriander powder, cayenne pepper, and cumin powder to a food processor. Process until the cilantro and parsley leaves are coarsely chopped.
3. Now add the saffron and lemon juice. Pulse until well-combined.
4. Turn on the food processor and slowly add the olive oil while the processor is running. Process until the sauce is smooth and creamy. Sprinkle with kosher salt and give the sauce a stir. The chermoula is ready.
5. Take a large glass bowl and place the beets into the same. Pour the chermoula sauce over the beets and mix until they are well-coated.
6. Take out the air fryer basket and place the coated beets into the same. Cook for about 30 minutes at 380°F.
7. Transfer the air-fried beets into a serving bowl and garnish with parsley and cilantro.

Crispy Buffalo Cauliflower

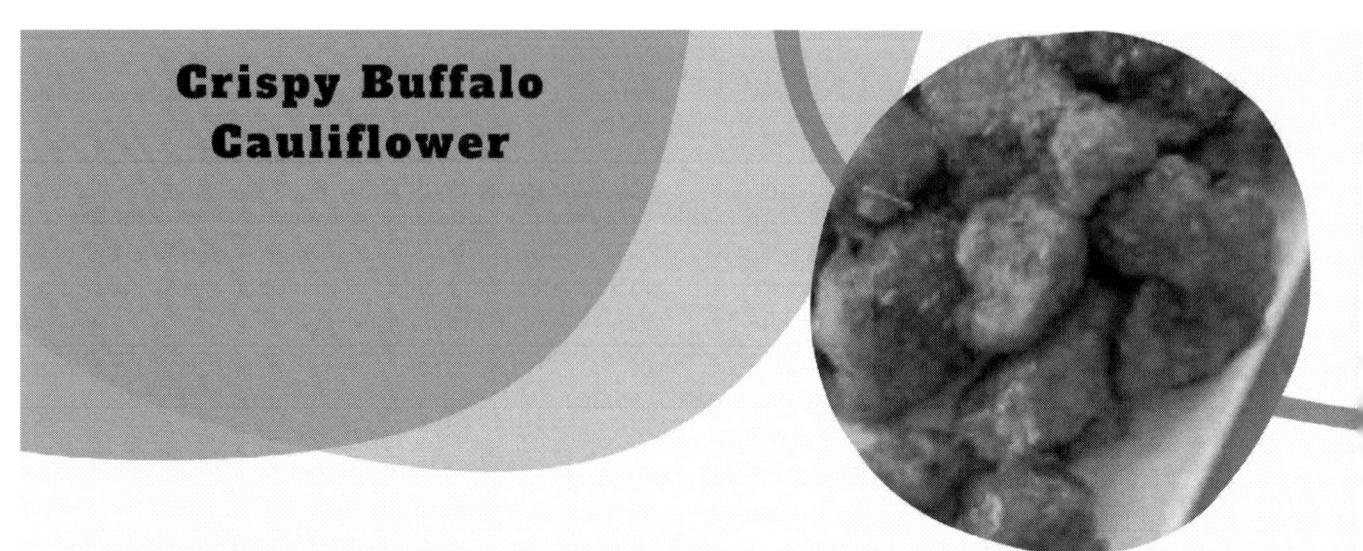

GENERAL INFO

Serving Size: 1
Servings per Recipe: 1
Calories: 101 calories per serving
Total Time: 20 minutes

INGREDIENTS

Cauliflower – 1 head
Olive oil spray
Buffalo sauce – ½ cup
Butter (melted) – 1 tablespoon
Salt – as per taste
Pepper – as per taste

NUTRITION INFO

Fat – 7 g
Protein – 3 g
Carbohydrates – 4 g

Crispy Buffalo Cauliflower

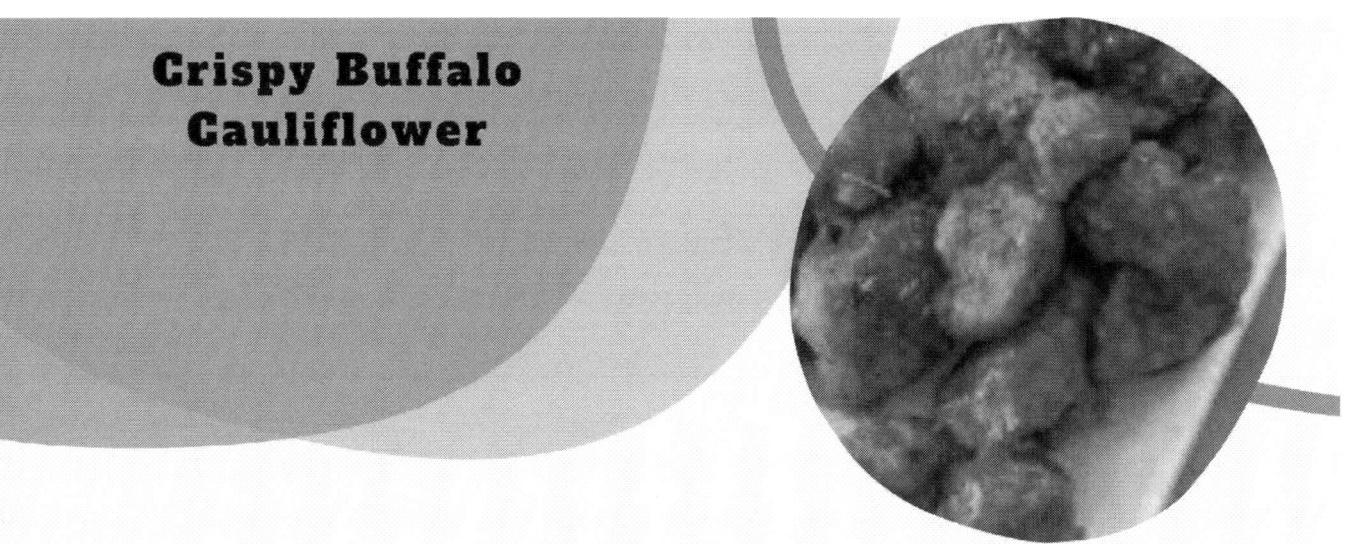

DIRECTIONS

1. Start by cutting the cauliflower head into bite-size pieces.
2. Grease the air-fry basket with olive oil spray.
3. Place the cauliflower pieces into the air fryer basket and lightly grease using olive oil spray. Let them cook for about 7 minutes at 400°F.
4. Take a bowl and add the buffalo sauce, melted butter, pepper, and salt. Whisk well to combine.
5. Transfer the cauliflower from the air fryer basket to a large glass bowl. Pour the prepared sauce over the cauliflower florets and mix well. Ensure all the florets are perfectly coated.
6. Transfer the coated cauliflower to the air fryer basket and cook for another 7 minutes at 400°F.
7. Transfer the cooked cauliflower onto a serving platter. Serve hot with the dip of your choice.

Crisped Tofu in an Air Fryer

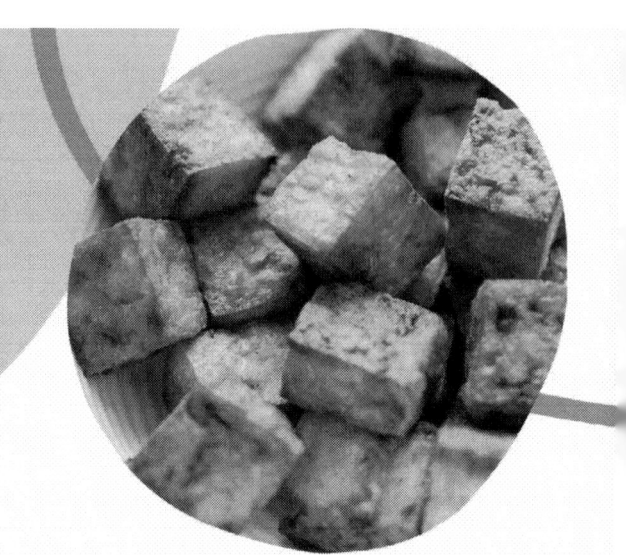

GENERAL INFO

Serving Size: 1
Servings per Recipe: 4
Calories: 63 calories per serving
Total Time: 15 minutes

INGREDIENTS

Extra-firm tofu – 14 ounces
Cornstarch – 1 tablespoon
Smoked paprika – 1 teaspoon
Coriander powder – ½ teaspoon
Sea salt – as per taste

NUTRITION INFO

Fat – 1 g
Protein – 7 g
Carbohydrates – 4 g

Crisped Tofu in an Air Fryer

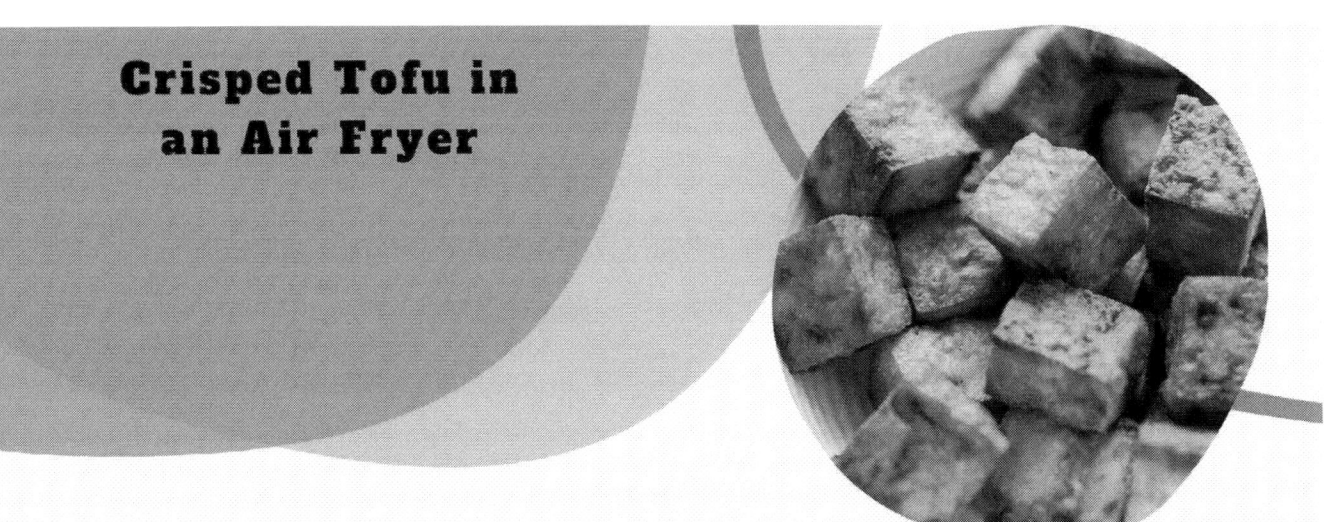

DIRECTIONS

1. Start by turning on the air fryer and setting the temperature to 375°F.
2. Take a bowl and add the cornstarch, smoked paprika, salt, and coriander powder. Mix well to combine.
3. Place the tofu on a wooden chopping block and cut it into rectangular cubes.
4. Take a zip-lock bag and add the tofu and cornstarch mixture. Shake well until the tofu pieces are evenly coated.
5. Place the coated tofu pieces into the air fryer basket and let them cook for about 6 minutes. Flip over and cook for another 6 minutes.
6. Transfer onto a platter and serve with the dip of your choice.

Easy-Peasy Ratatouille

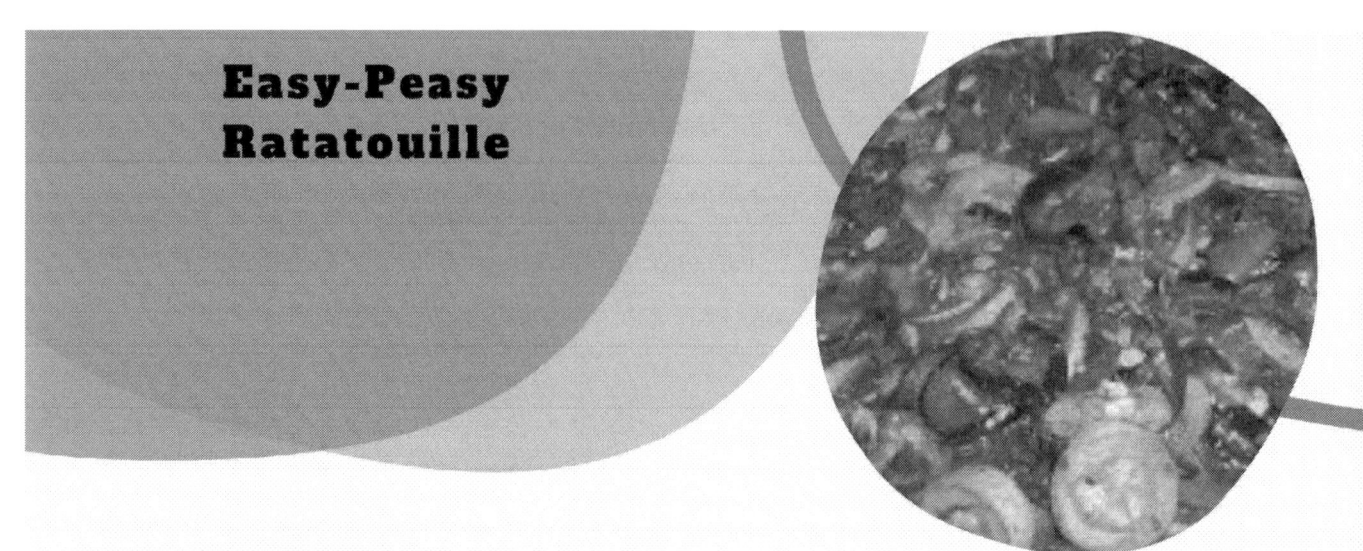

GENERAL INFO

Serving Size: 1
Servings per Recipe: 2
Calories: 238 calories per serving
Total Time: 50 minutes

INGREDIENTS

Eggplant – 2 cups
Sweet bell peppers – 1 cup
Cherry tomatoes – 1 cup
Garlic – 6-8 cloves
Oil – 3 tablespoons
Dried oregano – 1 teaspoon
Salt – 1 teaspoon
Black pepper (freshly ground) – ½ teaspoon
Dried thyme – ½ teaspoon

NUTRITION INFO

Fat – 21 g
Protein – 2 g
Carbohydrates – 12 g

Easy-Peasy Ratatouille

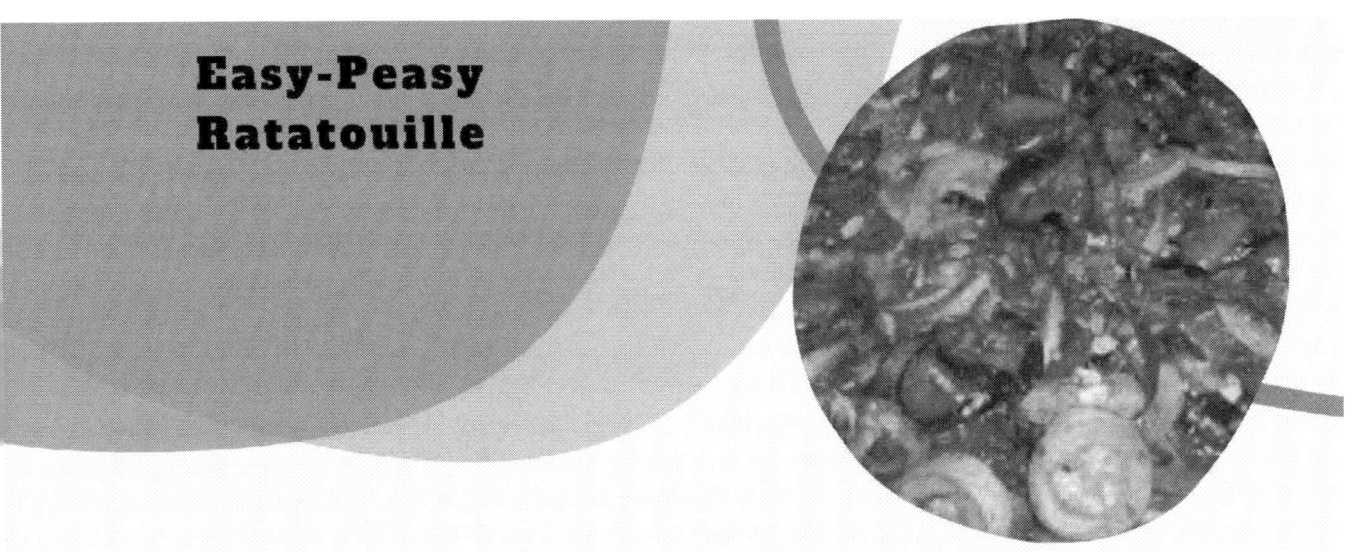

DIRECTIONS

1. Start by peeling the eggplant. Now dice both the sweet bell pepper and peeled eggplant into cubes (measuring ¾ inch).
2. Take a medium-sized glass bowl and add the bell peppers, eggplant, garlic, tomatoes, salt, thyme, pepper, oregano, and oil. Mix well until all the vegetables are evenly coated.
3. Place the coated vegetables into the air fryer basket and let them cook for 20 minutes at 400°F.
4. The veggies should be tender by now and reduced to half
5. Serve hot as a man dish or pair it with a side dish.

Healthy Brussels Sprouts

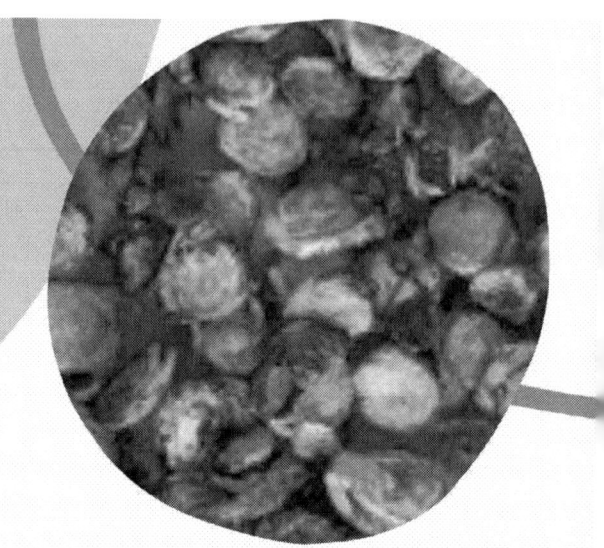

GENERAL INFO

Serving Size: 1
Servings per Recipe: 4
Calories: 155 calories per serving
Total Time: 20 minutes

INGREDIENTS

Brussels sprouts – 2 cups
Coconut oil – 2 tablespoons
Parmesan cheese (grated) – ¼ cup
Almonds (sliced) – ¼ cup
Everything bagel seasoning – 2 tablespoons
Sea salt – as per taste

NUTRITION INFO

Fat – 13 g
Protein – 6 g
Carbohydrates – 6 g

Healthy Brussels Sprouts

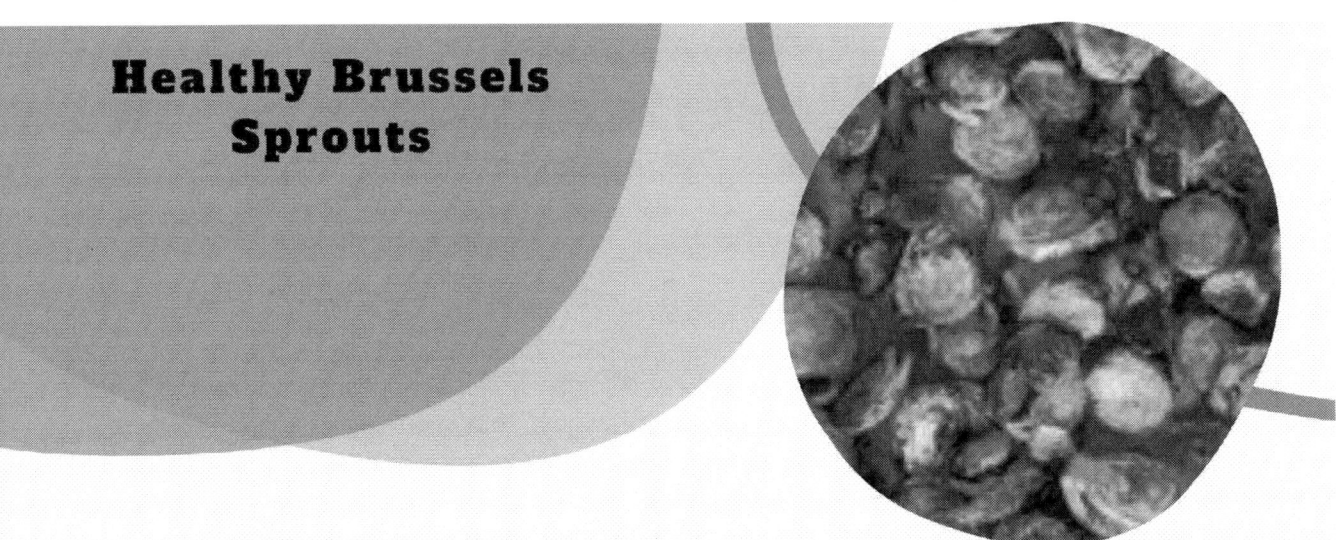

DIRECTIONS

1. Begin by placing a medium saucepan over a medium flame. Add about 2 cups of water and let it come to a boil.
2. Once the water starts boiling, add the Brussels sprouts and cook for about 10 minutes.
3. Once done, drain the Brussels and set aside to let them cook. Slice each Brussels sprout into 2 equal halves.
4. Toss the Brussels sprouts into a large glass mixing bowl and add the parmesan cheese, sliced almonds, salt, oil, and everything bagel seasoning. Mix well until the Brussels sprouts are evenly coated.
5. Place the Brussels sprouts into the air fryer basket and let them cook for about 15 minutes at 375°F. Serve hot!

Low-Carb Lebanese Muhammara

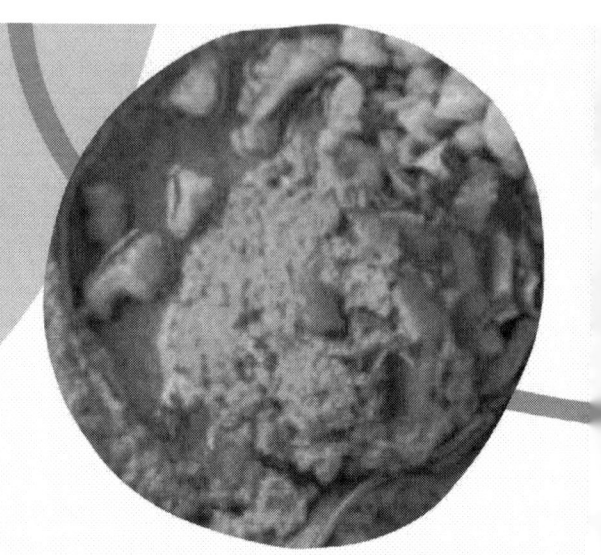

GENERAL INFO

Serving Size: 1
Servings per Recipe: 4
Calories: 272 calories per serving
Total Time: 25 minutes

INGREDIENTS

Red bell peppers – 2 large
Walnuts – 1 cup
Lemon juice – 1 teaspoon
Ground cumin – 1 teaspoon
Salt – 1 teaspoon
Red pepper flakes – 1 teaspoon
Olive oil – ¼ cup
Olive oil spray

NUTRITION INFO

Fat – 26 g
Protein – 3 g
Carbohydrates – 6 g

Low-Carb Lebanese Muhammara

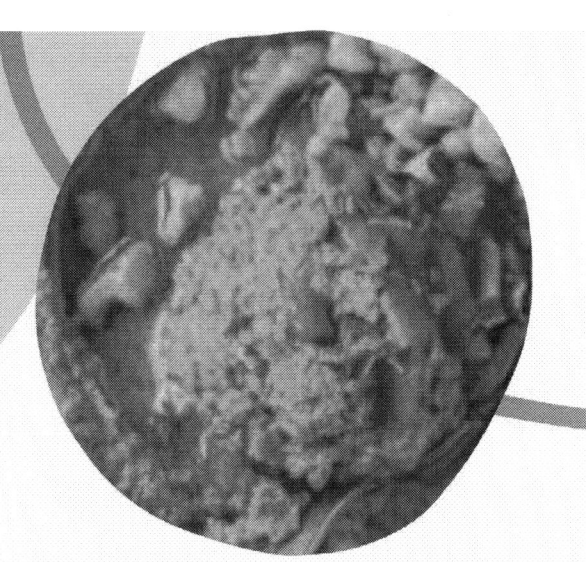

DIRECTIONS

1. Start by spraying the red peppers with olive oil spray.
2. Place the peppers in the basket of the air fryer and cook for 10 minutes at 400°F.
3. Once done, add the walnuts to the basket and air-fry for another 5 minutes.
4. Transfer the peppers to a zip-lock bag and let them sit for about 10 minutes. This will allow them to soften.
5. In a food processor bowl, add the softened peppers, lemon juice, walnuts, cumin, ½ teaspoon of pepper flakes, and salt. Process until smooth.
6. Transfer the puree into a bowl. Make a well in the middle and pour in the olive oil.
7. Finish by sprinkling pepper flakes on top.

Tip: This is best served with fresh vegetables like carrots, cucumbers, and zucchini.

Stuffed Cremini Mushrooms

GENERAL INFO

Serving Size: 1
Servings per Recipe: 6
Calories: 41 calories per serving
Total Time: 27 minutes

NUTRITION INFO

Fat – 3 g
Protein – 3 g
Carbohydrates – 2 g

INGREDIENTS

Cremini mushrooms – 14
Olive oil – 1 teaspoon
Salt – ⅛ teaspoon
Black pepper (crushed) – ⅛ teaspoon
Balsamic vinegar – 1 teaspoon

Filling
Bell pepper – ¼ cup
Onion (chopped) – ¼ cup
Cilantro (chopped) – 2 tablespoons
Jalapeno (finely chopped) – 1 tablespoon
Mozzarella cheese (shredded) – ⅓-½ cup grated
Ground coriander – 1 teaspoon
Salt – ¼ teaspoon
Paprika – ¼ teaspoon

Stuffed Cremini Mushrooms

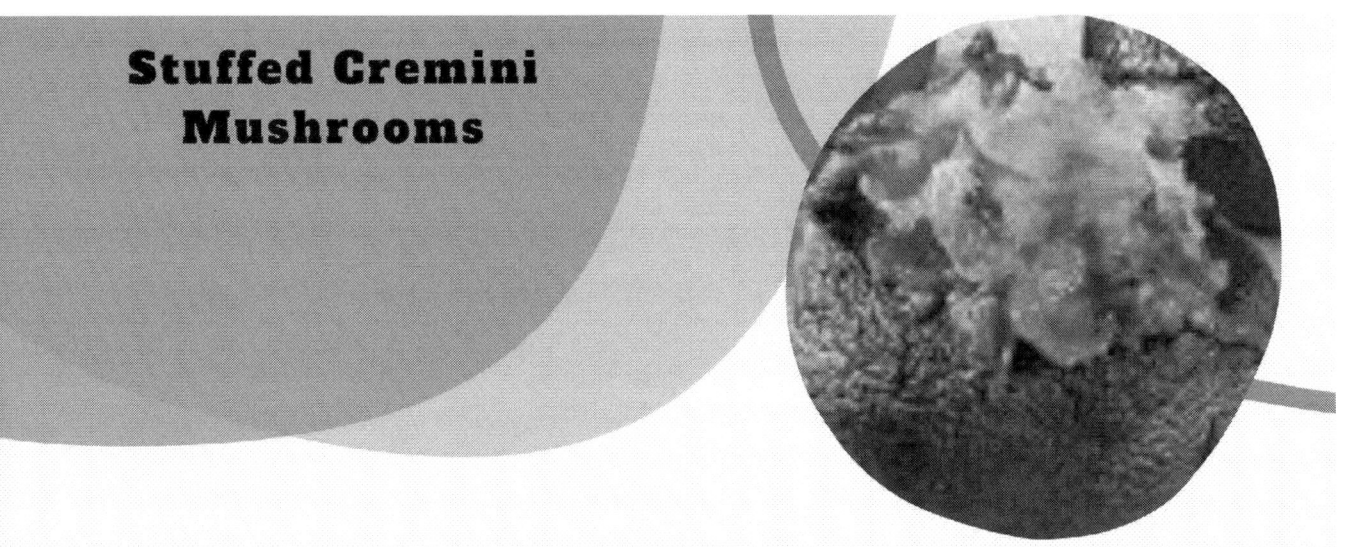

DIRECTIONS

1. Begin by cleaning the mushrooms with a damp cloth. Remove the stems by pulling them sideways.
2. Season the mushrooms. For this, toss the mushrooms into a large bowl and add the olive oil, black pepper, balsamic vinegar, and salt. Mix until well-coated.
3. Take another bowl and add the chopped pepper, jalapeno, onion, cilantro, ground coriander, salt, paprika, and shredded cheese. Mix well.
4. Place the mushrooms on a large plate and stuff the cremini mushrooms caps with 1 teaspoon of filling.
5. Place the stuffed cremini mushrooms into the air fryer basket and cook for 10 minutes at 320°F.
6. Transfer onto a serving platter and serve with the dip of your choice.

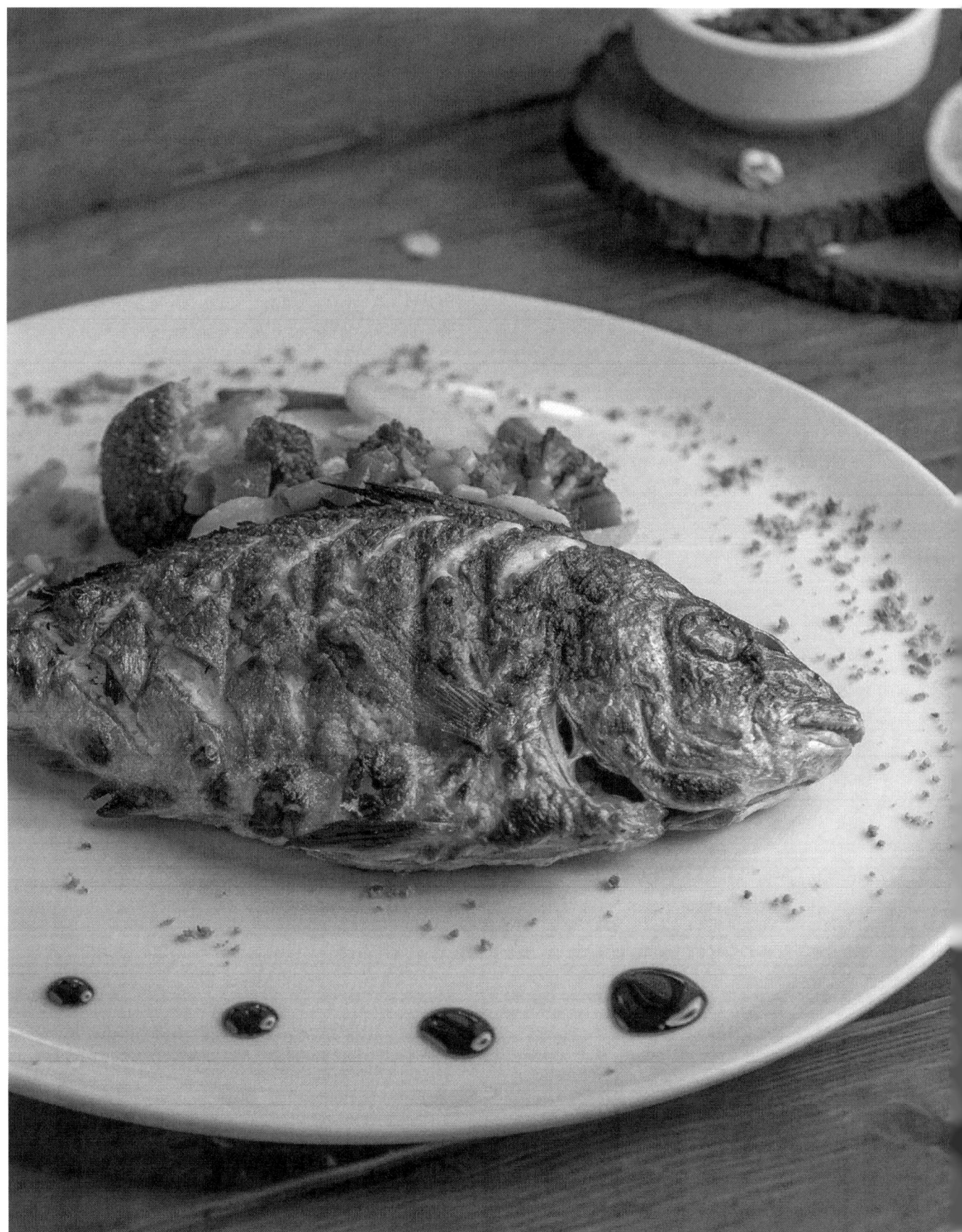

seafood
RECIPES

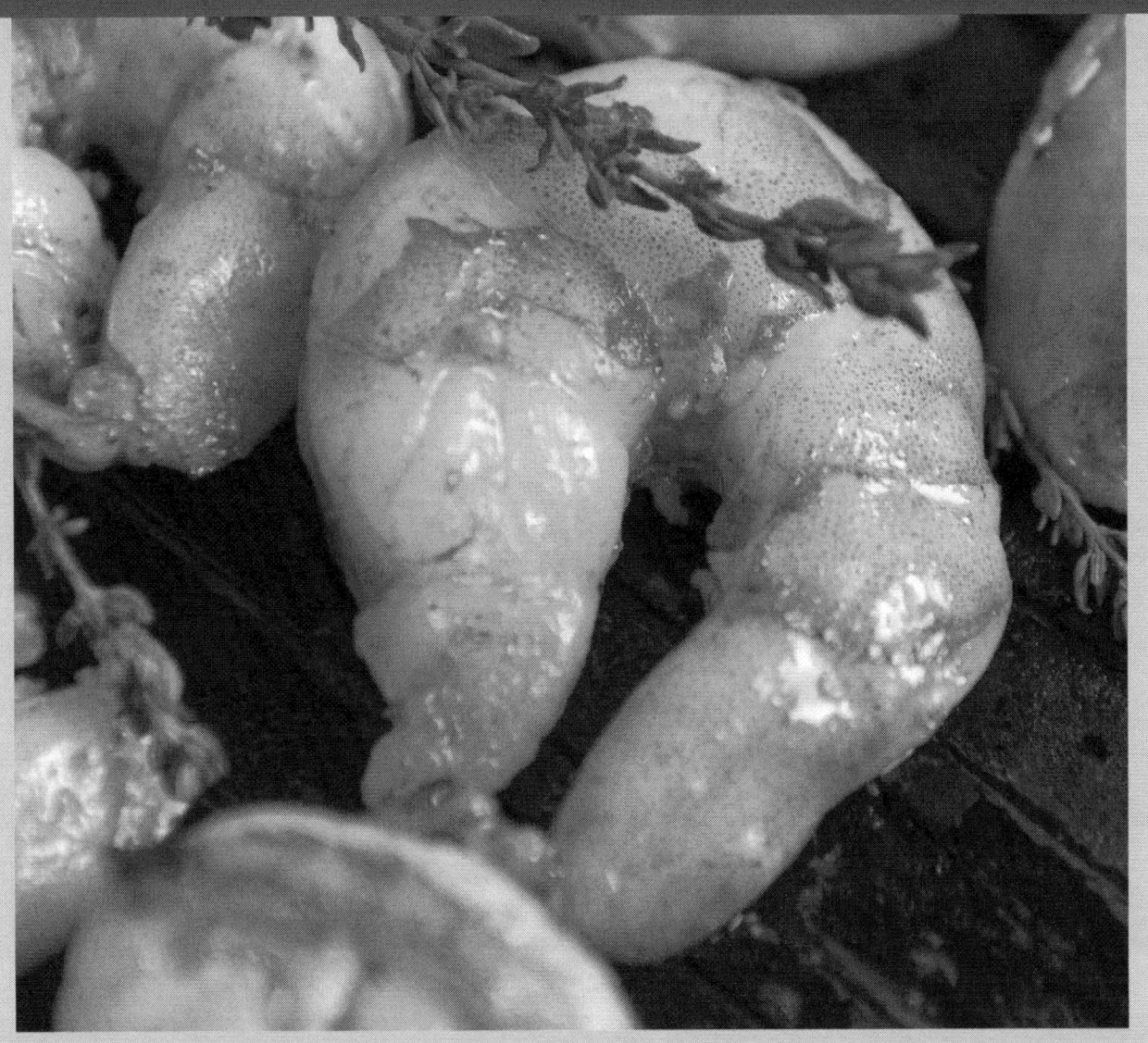

Air Fryer Fish En Papillote

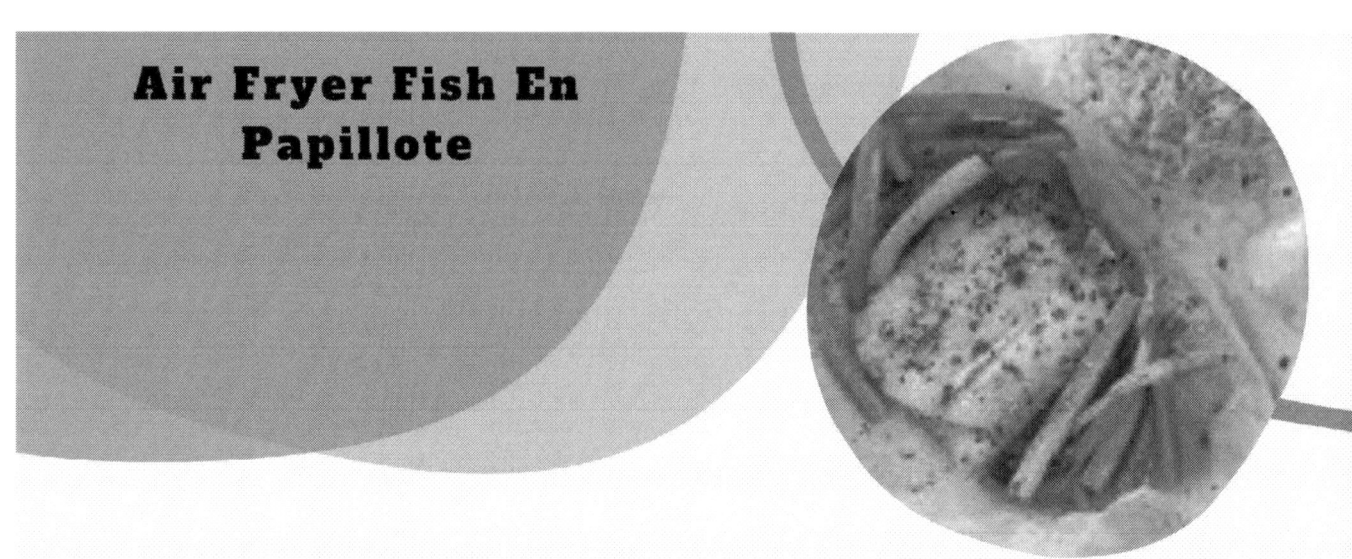

GENERAL INFO

Serving Size: 1
Servings per Recipe: 2
Calories: 251 calories per serving
Total Time: 25 minutes

INGREDIENTS

Cod fillets (thawed) – 2
Carrots (julienned) – ½ cup
Fennel bulbs (julienned) – ½ cup
Red peppers (thinly sliced) – ½ cup
Tarragon – 2 sprigs
Butter (melted) – 2 pats
Lemon juice – 1 tablespoon
Salt (divided) – 1 tablespoon
Black pepper (freshly ground) – ½ teaspoon
Olive oil – 1 tablespoon
Olive oil spray

NUTRITION INFO

Fat – 12 g
Protein – 26 g
Carbohydrates – 8 g

Air Fryer Fish En Papillote

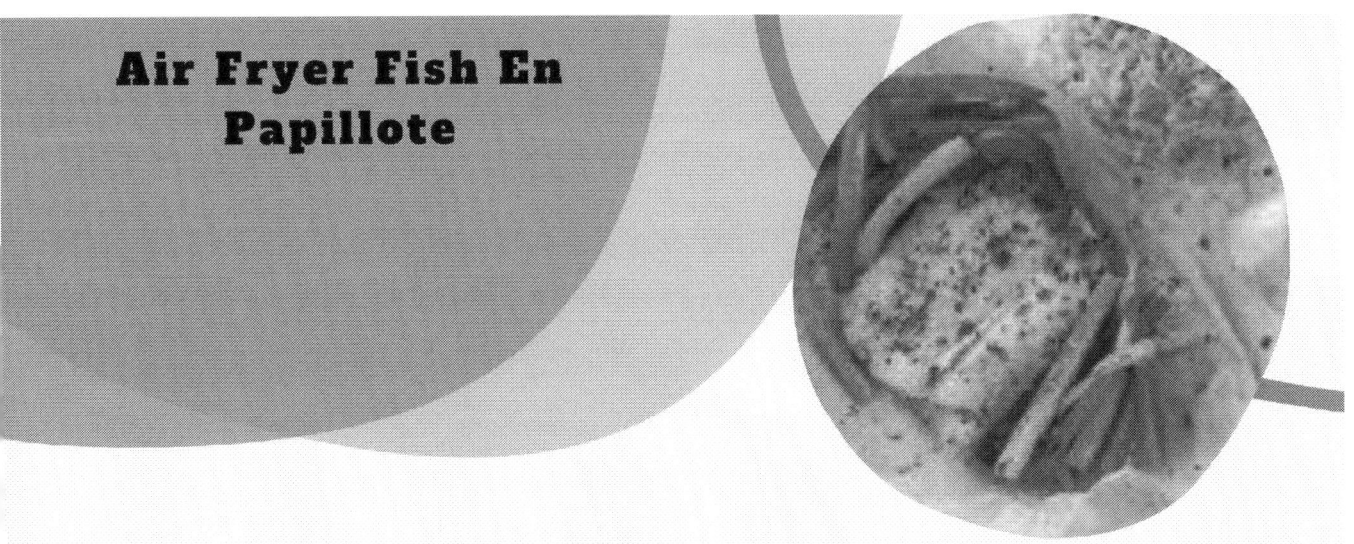

DIRECTIONS

1. Take a glass mixing bowl and add the butter, ½ teaspoon of salt, lemon juice, and tarragon. Whisk until smooth.
2. Add the carrots, red peppers, and fennel bulbs and mix well. Set aside.
3. Take 2 large parchment sheets and cut them into equal-sized squares.
4. Place the fish fillets on a plate and grease them with olive oil spray.
5. Take the parchment sheet squares and lay one fillet on each of the squares.
6. Top the fillets with the vegetable mixture. Any remaining sauce can be drizzled over the cod fillets.
7. Bring together all 4 edges of the parchment squares and enclose by crimping. Make sure the packet is properly sealed.
8. Take out the air fryer basket and place the prepared fillet packets into the same. Return the basket to the fryer.
9. Cook the fillets for 15 minutes at 350°F.
10. Once done, transfer the ingredients of the packet onto a serving platter.
11. Serve hot immediately!

Air-Fried Shrimp Scampi

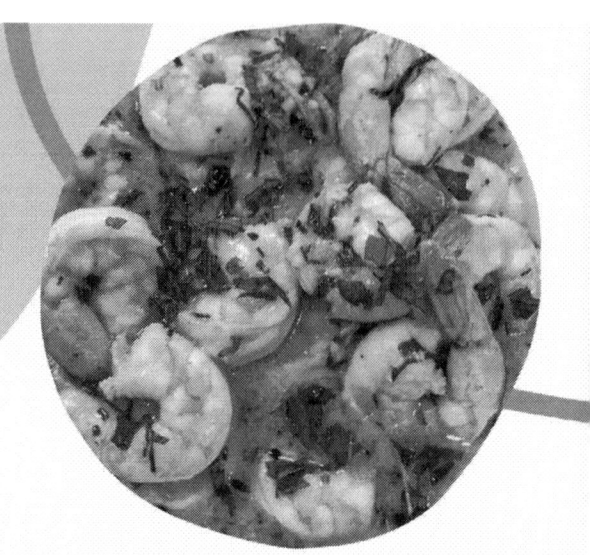

GENERAL INFO

Serving Size: 1
Servings per Recipe: 4
Calories: 221 calories per serving
Total Time: 15 minutes

INGREDIENTS

Butter – 4 tablespoons
Lemon juice – 1 tablespoon
Garlic (minced) – 1 tablespoon
Red pepper flakes – 2 teaspoons
Chives (chopped) – 1 tablespoon
Fresh basil (chopped) – 1 tablespoon
Chicken stock – 2 tablespoons
Shrimp – 25 (about 1 pound)

NUTRITION INFO

Fat – 13 g
Protein – 23 g
Carbohydrates – 1 g

Air-Fried Shrimp Scampi

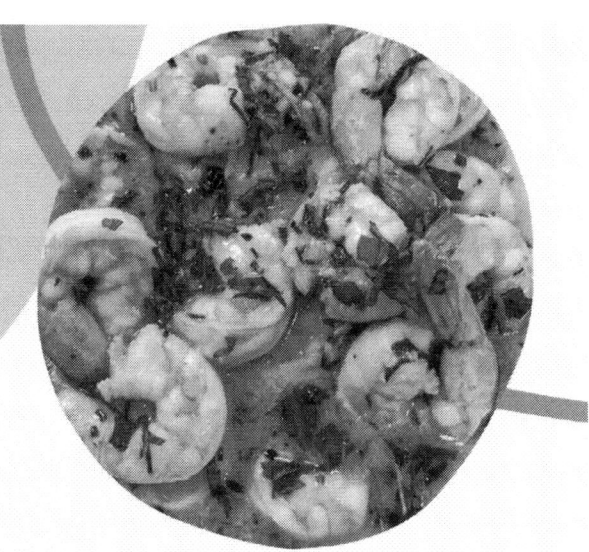

DIRECTIONS

1. Start by preheating the air fryer at 330°F. Place a tin pan into the basket and let it preheat as well.
2. Open the basket and add the butter, red pepper flakes, and garlic. Let the ingredients cook for a couple of minutes. This will help infuse flavor into the butter.
3. Once done, add the lemon juice, chives, chicken stock, and shrimps. Stir well. (Cook in batches, if required.)
4. Return the basket to the air fryer and let the shrimps in herb sauce cook for about 5 minutes.
5. Remove the shrimps from the air fryer and let them rest for a few minutes.
6. Give them a nice stir and transfer into a serving bowl.
7. Finish by garnishing with chopped fresh basil leaves.

Cheesy Crab Dip

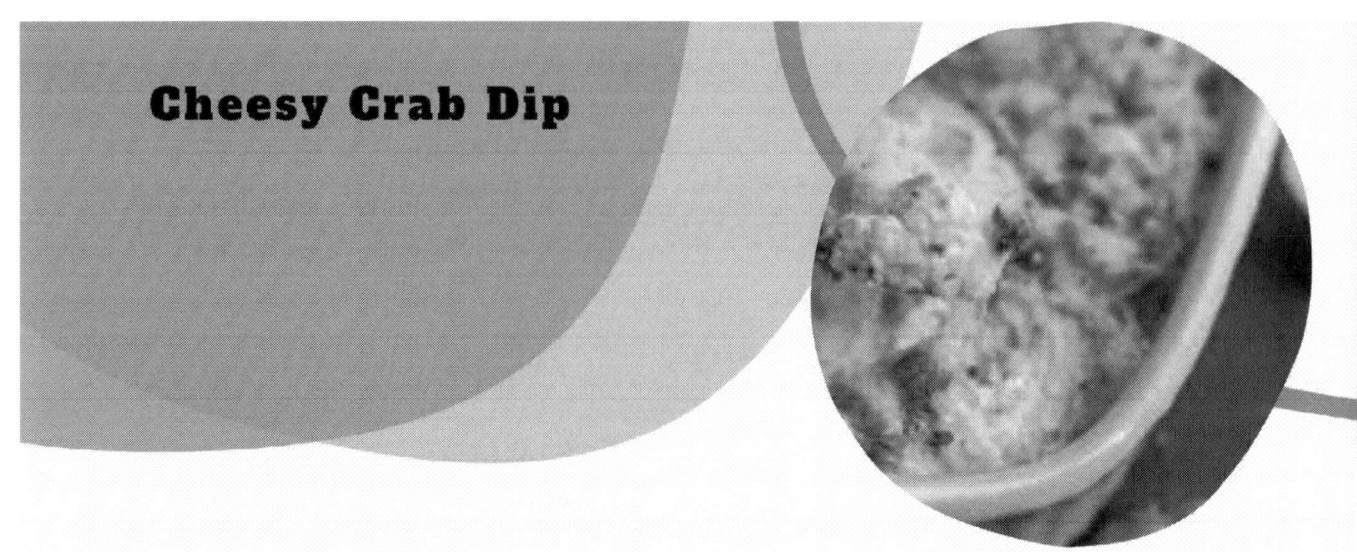

GENERAL INFO

Serving Size: 1
Servings per Recipe: 4
Calories: 359 calories per serving
Total Time: 12 minutes

INGREDIENTS

Crab (cooked) – 1 cup
Mayonnaise – ¼ cup
Jalapeno jack cheese (grated) – 2 cups
Scallions – ½ cup
Hot sauce – 2 tablespoons
Salt – ½ teaspoon
Black pepper (freshly ground) – 1 teaspoon
Lemon juice – 2 tablespoons
Parsley (chopped) – 2 tablespoons

NUTRITION INFO

Fat – 29 g
Protein – 20 g
Carbohydrates – 1 g

Cheesy Crab Dip

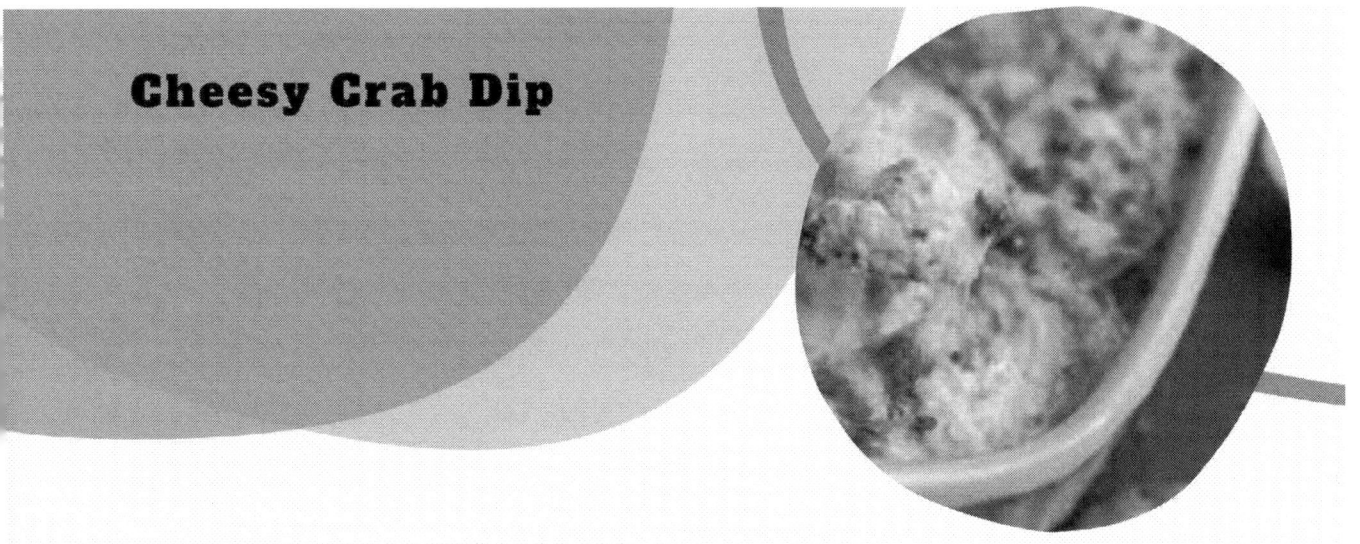

DIRECTIONS

1. Take a tin pan that fits into the air fryer basket and add the crab, cheese, mayonnaise, salt, pepper, scallions, and hot sauce. Mix well to combine.
2. Place the tin pan into the basket of the air fryer.
3. Let the crabs cook for about 7 minutes at 400°F.
4. Remove the tin pan from the air fryer and add the parsley and lemon juice.
5. Serve hot!

Healthy Niçoise Salad

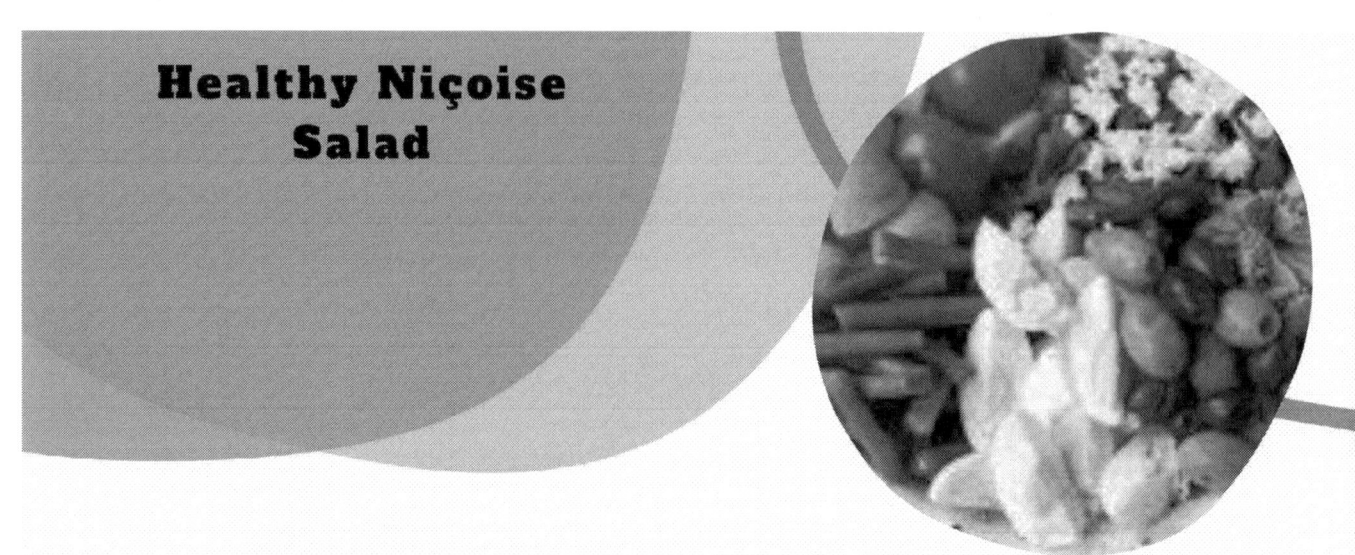

GENERAL INFO

Serving Size: 1
Servings per Recipe: 2
Calories: 601 calories per serving
Total Time: 35 minutes

NUTRITION INFO

Fat – 27 g
Protein – 41 g
Carbohydrates –48 g

INGREDIENTS

New baby potatoes (quartered) – 6
Vegetable oil – 2 teaspoons
Olive oil spray
Salt – as per taste
Black pepper (ground) – as per taste
Green beans (trim and snap in half) – 1 cup
Tuna fillets – 2 (4 ounces each)
Cherry tomatoes – 1 cup
Butter lettuce – 6 leaves
Hard-boiled eggs (peel and cut in half) – 2
Olives – 10

Vinaigrette Dressing
Olive oil – 2 tablespoons
Red wine vinegar – 1 tablespoon
Salt – ⅛ teaspoon
Dijon mustard – 1 teaspoon
Black pepper (freshly ground) – as per taste

Healthy Niçoise Salad

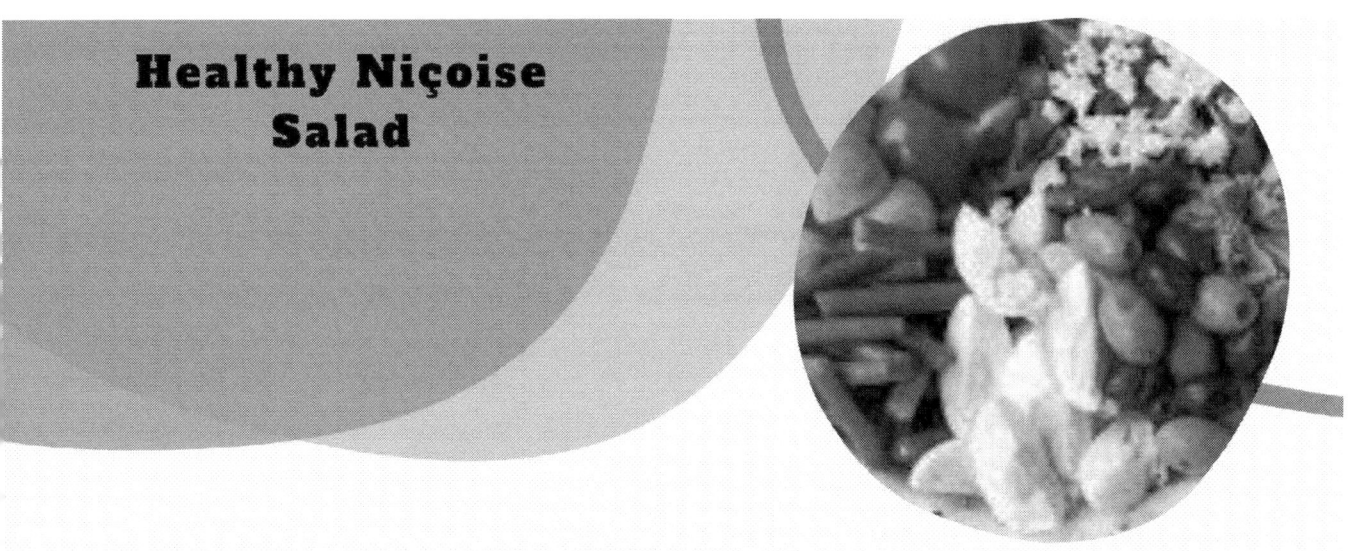

DIRECTIONS

1. Start by tossing the potatoes, beans, tomatoes, salt, pepper, and 2 teaspoons of vegetable oil in a mixing bowl.
2. Take the basket out of the air fryer and place the seasoned vegetables in the same. Make sure to arrange the vegetables in a single layer.
3. Return the basket to the fryer and cook for about 10 minutes at 400°F.
4. Grease both sides of the tuna fillets with olive oil spray. Generously season the fish with pepper and salt.
5. Take out the air fryer basket and place the fillets over the vegetables. Let them cook for about 5 minutes. The tuna should be medium-well by now.
6. Remove the tuna and set it aside for a few minutes. Cut into slices.
7. Meanwhile, prepare the vinaigrette. For this, add the vinegar, mustard, salt, black pepper, and olive oil to a small glass jar and close the lid. Shake until well-combined.
8. Place the butter lettuce leaves on a flat wooden surface and place equal amounts of tuna, tomatoes, potatoes, and green beans on the lettuce leaves.
9. Take 2 serving platters and place 3 prepared lettuce salad bowls on each platter.
10. Place 2 egg halves on each of the serving platters and sprinkle with chopped olives.
11. Finish by drizzling vinaigrette on top of all the salad bowls. Serve fresh!

Low-Carb Bok Choy Salmon

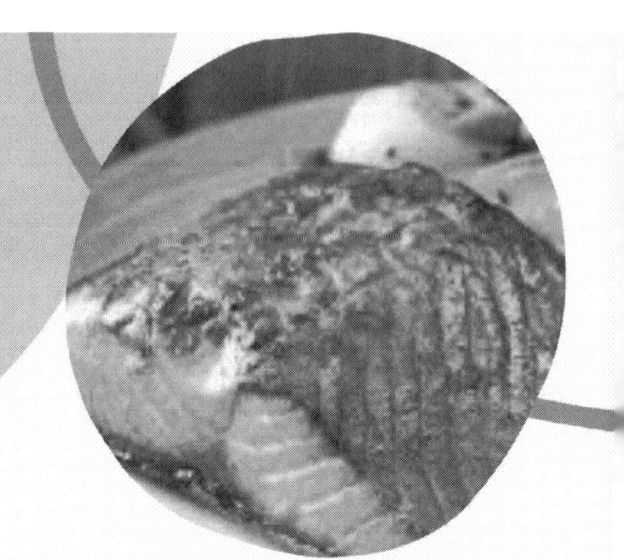

GENERAL INFO

Serving Size: 1
Servings per Recipe: 2
Calories: 195 calories per serving
Total Time: 1 hour 2 minutes

INGREDIENTS

Garlic (minced) – 2 cloves
Ginger (minced) – 1 tablespoon
Orange zest (finely grated) – 2 teaspoons
Fresh orange juice – ½ cup
Soy sauce – ¼ cup
Rice vinegar – 3 tablespoons
Vegetable oil – 1 tablespoon
Salt – ½ teaspoon
Salmon fillets – 2 (5 ounces)

For the vegetables
Baby bok choy – 2 heads
Shiitake mushrooms – 2 ounces
Dark sesame oil – 1 tablespoon
Salt – as per taste
Sesame seeds (toasted) – ½ teaspoon

NUTRITION INFO

Fat – 14 g
Protein – 4 g
Carbohydrates – 12 g

Low-Carb Bok Choy Salmon

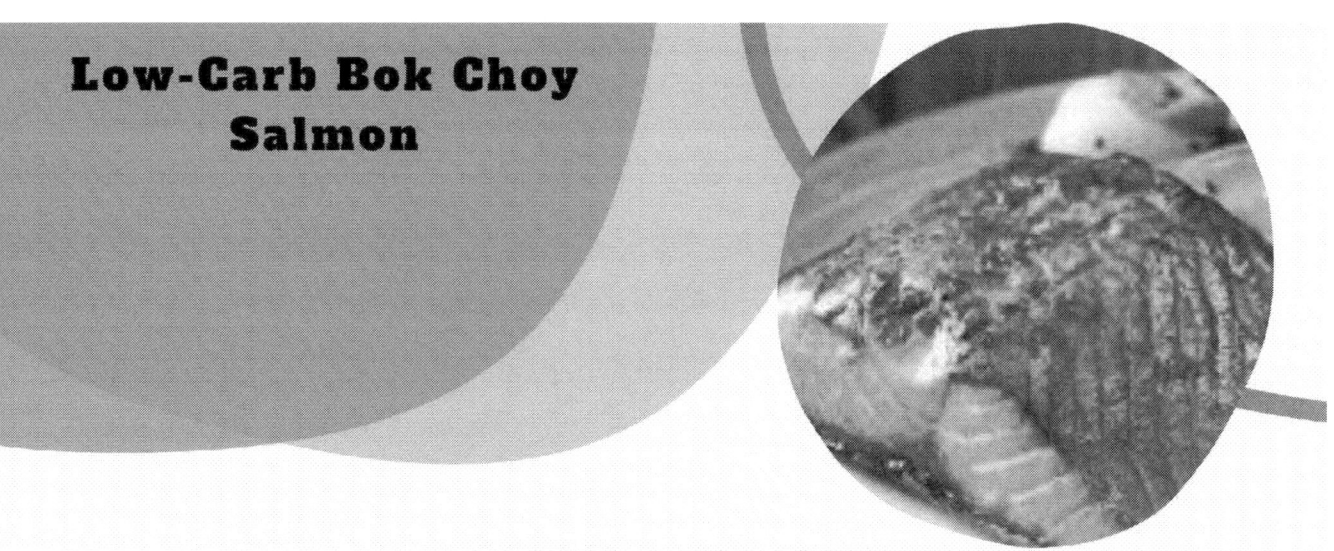

DIRECTIONS

1. Start by cutting the bok choy into half lengthwise. Also, remove the stems from the shiitake mushrooms. Set aside.
2. Prepare the fish marinade. For this, take a glass bowl and add the ginger, garlic, orange juice, orange zest, vegetable oil, salt, vinegar, and soy sauce. Mix well.
3. Take a large zip-lock bag and place the salmon fillets inside the same. Pour half of the marinade into the zip-lock bag and let the fillets marinate for about 30 minutes at room temperature. Save the remaining marinade for later.
4. Once the fish is done marinating, place the fillets into the basket and return to the air fryer.
5. Cook the fish fillets for 6 minutes at 400°F.
6. While the fish is cooking, brush the mushroom caps and bok choy with dark sesame oil. Nicely season the vegetables with salt.
7. After 6 minutes, take out the air fryer basket and add the vegetables. Cook for another 6 minutes.
8. Transfer the cooked salmon onto a serving platter and drizzle with the remaining marinade.
9. Place the cooked veggies alongside the salmon and finish by sprinkling with sesame seeds.

Scallops in Creamy Tomato Basil Sauce

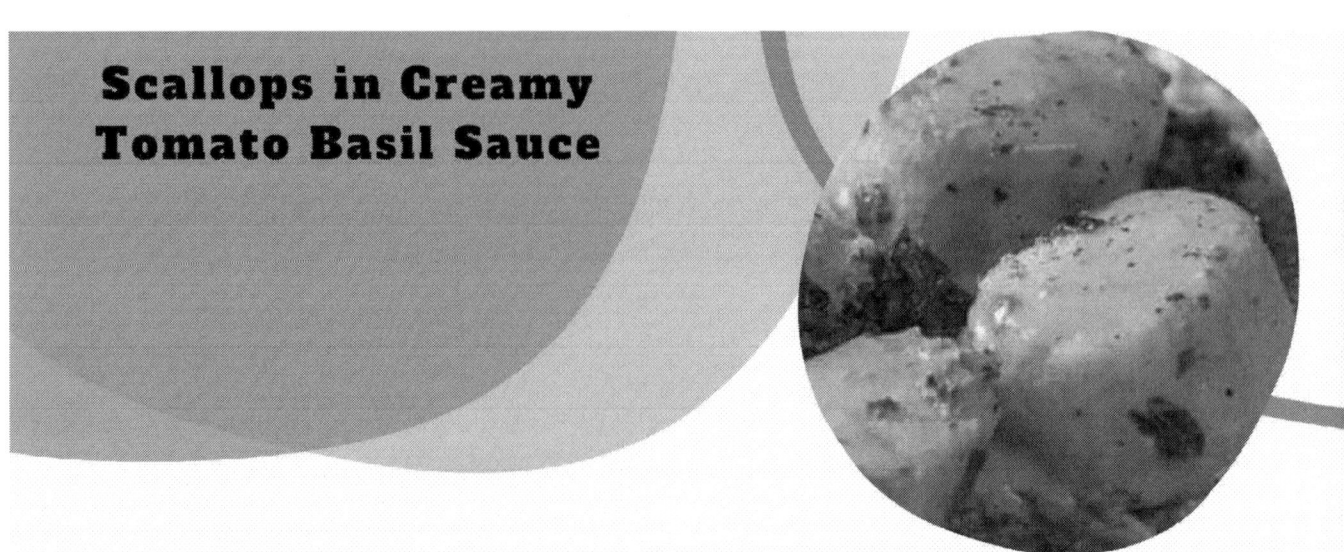

GENERAL INFO

Serving Size: 1
Servings per Recipe: 2
Calories: 359 calories per serving
Total Time: 15 minutes

INGREDIENTS

Heavy whipping cream – ¾ cup
Tomato paste – 1 tablespoon
Fresh basil (chopped) – 1 tablespoon
Garlic (minced) – 1 teaspoon
Salt – ½ teaspoon
Ground black pepper – ½ teaspoon
Frozen spinach (thaw and drain) – 12 ounces
Jumbo sea scallops – 8
Cooking oil spray
Salt – for seasoning
Pepper – for seasoning

NUTRITION INFO

Fat – 33 g
Protein – 9 g
Carbohydrates – 6 g

Scallops in Creamy Tomato Basil Sauce

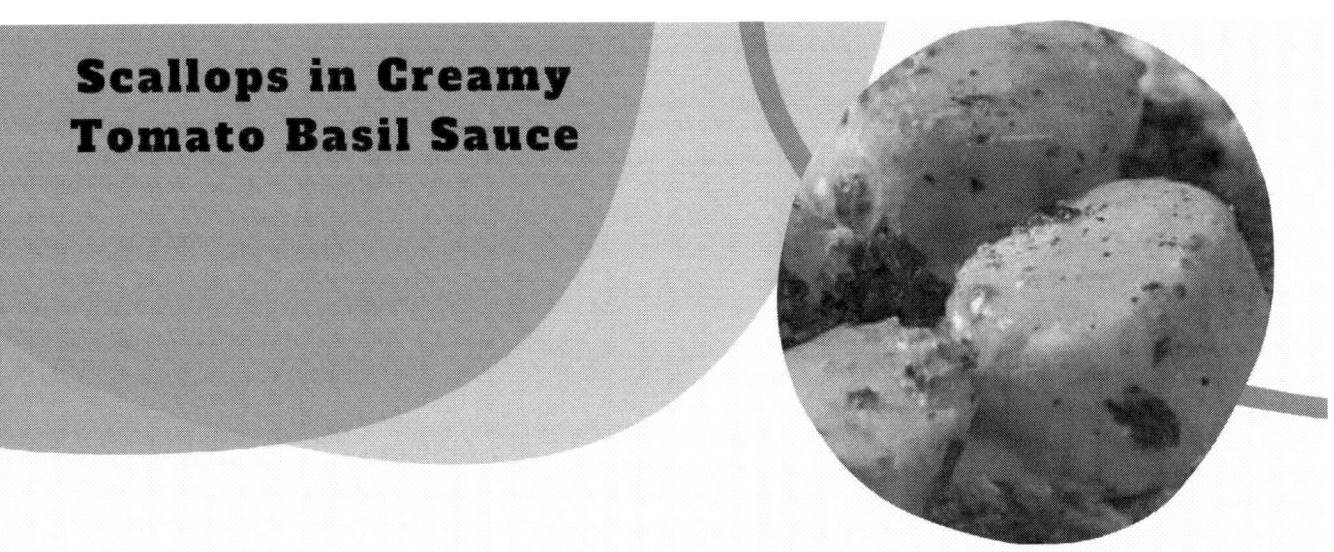

DIRECTIONS

1. Start by greasing a tin pan using the cooking oil spray. Layer the bottom of the pan with spinach.
2. Also, grease the scallops with oil spray. Now season the scallops with pepper and salt.
3. Place the scallops over the spinach. Make sure they do not overlap each other.
4. Take a small glass bowl and add the cream, basil, tomato paste, salt, pepper, and garlic. Mix well to combine.
5. Pour the prepared creamy tomato and basil sauce over the scallops and spinach.
6. Place the tin pan into the air fryer basket and cook for 10 minutes at 350°F.
7. Serve hot!

An Appeal from the Publisher

Hello wonderful reader!

We hope you are enjoying this book.

We wanted to let you know that you have made an impact on many lives by purchasing this book.

Just to give you a brief introduction: We are a small publishing company with a team of 8 writers and 2 editors.

Most of our employees come from financially weaker section and our company is the only means they support their families. This is our way of giving back to the society.

We don't have the giant advertising budgets that many other publishers and businesses do online.

So, one way that you can really support our mission and our business is by leaving us a review on this book.

For a small company like us, getting reviews (especially on Amazon) means we can submit our books for advertising.

This means we can actually sell a few copies from time to time and make a bigger impact on the society as a whole. So, every review means a lot to us.

We can't THANK YOU enough for this!

Thank you so much

Manufactured by Amazon.ca
Bolton, ON